Righting Health Policy

REVOLUTIONARY BIOETHICS

Series Editor: Rachel Haliburton, University of Sudbury

Revolutionary Bioethics is a new series composed of scholarly monographs and edited collections organized around specific topics that explore bioethical theory and practice through the frameworks provided by feminist ethics, narrative ethics, and virtue ethics, challenging the assumptions of mainstream bioethics in the process. Contemporary mainstream bioethics has become ideological and repetitive, a defender of activities that bioethics was originally created to critique, and an apologist for unethical practices and policies in medicine that it once saw itself as fighting against. Taking its title from recent work being done on MacIntyre's neo-Aristotelian ethics, Revolutionary Bioethics is organized around the idea that bioethics needs to reform both its theory and practice, and its goal is to begin the conversation about what a transformed bioethics—one that is unafraid to explore new theoretical approaches, and to examine and critique current bioethical practices—might look like.

Titles in the series

Righting Health Policy: Bioethics, Political Philosophy, and the Normative Justification of Health Law and Policy, by D. Robert MacDougall
Caregiving, Carebots, and Contagion, by Michael C. Brannigan
Engineering Perfection: Solidarity, Disability, and Well-being, by Elyse Purcell
Physician-Assisted Suicide and Euthanasia: Before, During, and After the Third Reich, Edited by Sheldon Rubenfeld and Daniel P. Sulmasy, with Astrid Ley

Righting Health Policy

Bioethics, Political Philosophy, and the Normative Justification of Health Law and Policy

D. Robert MacDougall

LEXINGTON BOOKS
Lanham • Boulder • New York • London

Published by Lexington Books
An imprint of The Rowman & Littlefield Publishing Group, Inc.
4501 Forbes Boulevard, Suite 200, Lanham, Maryland 20706
www.rowman.com

86-90 Paul Street, London EC2A 4NE

Copyright © 2022 by The Rowman & Littlefield Publishing Group, Inc.

All rights reserved. No part of this book may be reproduced in any form or by any electronic or mechanical means, including information storage and retrieval systems, without written permission from the publisher, except by a reviewer who may quote passages in a review.

British Library Cataloguing in Publication Information Available

Library of Congress Cataloging-in-Publication Data Available

ISBN 9781498589956 (cloth) | ISBN 9781498589963 (epub) | ISBN 9781498589970 (paper)

Contents

Acknowledgments	vii
Introduction	1
Chapter 1: The Political Tasks of Bioethics	13
Chapter 2: Bioethics and Its Political Philosophy Problem	35
Chapter 3: Bioethicists on Kant and the Legalization of Organ Markets	63
Chapter 4: Kantian Moral Theory and the Problem of Political Legitimacy	87
Chapter 5: Rights as the Basis for Political Legitimacy	105
Chapter 6: State Authority and Morally Justifiable Coercion	129
Chapter 7: Kidney Markets and the Limits of Legitimacy	161
Chapter 8: Legal Standards of Informed Consent and the Authority of the State	185
Conclusion	209
Bibliography	217
Index	227
About the Author	235

Acknowledgments

I owe gratitude to many others for help and encouragement during the writing of this book.

Participants in the New York City Early Career Ethics Workshop deserve special thanks for comments and feedback on earlier drafts of several chapters. Sean Aas, Collin O'Neil, Travis Timmerman, Sari Kisilevsky, Jacob Sparks, Duncan Purves, Regina Rini, and Daniel Fogal all provided comments and discussion on various chapters. The group has been encouraging in ways that go far beyond the present manuscript.

Audiences at the American Philosophical Association, American Society for Bioethics and the Humanities, Canadian Bioethics Society, MANCEPT Workshops in Political Theory, Dalhousie University, and New York City College of Technology have provided valuable input on previous drafts and talks.

A variety of friends and colleagues have provided thoughtful comments and encouragement at different stages of the writing process, including Nathaniel Brown, Aaron Jaffe, Tim Krahn, and Jason Breen.

Many colleagues at New York City College of Technology have also contributed in one way or another to the writing of this book. Dean Justin Vazquez-Poritz and President Russ Hotzler have both provided generous support with their time and energy in helping me obtain books, pay for conference travel, and organize research meetings on campus. Department chairs Peter Parides and Jean Hillstrom helped encourage, organize, and facilitate various affairs relevant to the book.

The City University of New York provided generous support for completing the manuscript through a CUNY Book Completion Award. The Professional Staff Congress of the City University of New York provided grants that made it possible for me to spend three summers focusing on the present manuscript.

I owe an immense debt of gratitude to mentors who formed the intellectual communities in which I first began thinking about bioethics and political philosophy. I am particularly grateful to Griffin Trotter, Jeffrey Bishop, Francoise Baylis, Ana Iltis, and Tristram Engelhardt.

Editors Jana Hodges-Kluck and Rachel Halliburton at Lexington Books have been supportive and professional from our first interactions and have been gracious with me as I have tried to finish the manuscript through the midst of several moves, a wedding, and a global pandemic.

My parents have, together, been an unending source of encouragement and a dependable source for critical discussion of the themes in the book. My father, Dan MacDougall, gave me my first insight into the importance of scholarship and the possibility of contributing to a field by challenging widely held views. My mother, Barb MacDougall, has taught me the importance of communicating clearly. She contributed immensely to this book by reading the entire draft and providing copious editorial and critical comments.

Most important, I would like to thank Moby Halverson MacDougall, my wife, who has been the source of so much joy as I have been completing this manuscript."

Parts of chapters 3 and 7 appeared earlier as "Sometimes Merely as a Means: Why Kantian Philosophy Requires the Legalization of Kidney Sales." Copyright © 2019 Oxford University Press. This article first appeared in The Journal of Medicine and Philosophy Volume 44, no. 3 (2019), pages 314–34.

A version of chapter 8 first appeared as "Must Consent Be Informed? Patient Rights, State Authority, and the Moral Basis of the Physician's Duties of Disclosure." Copyright © 2021 Johns Hopkins University Press. This article first appeared in Kennedy Institute of Ethics Journal, volume 31, no. 3, 2021, pages 247–70.

Introduction

THE TASKS AND TOOLS OF BIOETHICS

There is an old saying that when you have a hammer, everything looks like a nail. It could mean that when you have a certain tool handy, it seems like the best tool for every task. Or, it could mean that when you have a tool, everything looks like a problem that needs to be fixed. Whatever else it means, though, it surely means that the tools we have at our disposal influence the way in which we solve problems. Sometimes we use a hammer when a pry bar, a mallet, or a nail puller would be better.

This is a book about tools, the tools that we use to judge the moral acceptability of laws and policies regulating health and the various practices of health care. What makes a law a good one? What makes a behavior deserving of regulation, incentivization, or prohibition? What should laws aim at? When do laws go too far? Answering these questions requires tools, or methods. It is crucially important that we use the right tool for the job when answering questions like these. I will argue that bioethics has not been using the right tools when answering questions such as these. It has tended to use the tools it has available rather than the best ones for the job.

The tools that I am primarily concerned with in this book are philosophical ones. The discussion about methods in bioethics is a relatively big and multifaceted one: bioethics is inherently interdisciplinary, and so there is no single set of tools applicable to all, or perhaps even *any*, bioethics problems or issues. Even the questions I listed above are not solely philosophical questions. When we ask whether a behavior should be regulated or prohibited, for example, sociology and the medical sciences might be relevant. In fact, it might be harder to list disciplines *not* relevant to these questions than it would be to make a list of those that are. Everything affects everything; how can any tool be the "wrong one" for the job, if we need so many tools to get a grasp on the moral problems we face in real life?

It would be foolish to bring only the tool you thought *most important* for a job to the task; you should bring a whole tool bag because for any problem, you may need more than one tool. Even so, there is often one or a small set of tools that are most important for the job at hand. My argument is, roughly, this: despite the large number of tools bioethics has brought to problems of health law and policy, it has generally failed to bring the most important one: political philosophy. The argument is about philosophical tools because I understand moral problems to be, at base, best answered by philosophical tools. These philosophical tools are commonly employed in the bioethics literature, where a significant percentage of the field is made up of professional philosophers. But the problem is that bioethicists have typically brought (to use another hackneyed saying) knives to a gunfight. They have used the principles, theories, and methods characteristic of moral philosophy when they should have been using political philosophy.[1] This has had a detrimental effect on the quality of the substantive answers bioethicists have given to normative questions surrounding health law and policy; and in many cases it has also caused debate to revolve around issues that are, I shall argue, not the most relevant to the problems for which they are thought foundational.

Defending these sweeping claims raises methodological problems of its own. Even if it were true, that bioethics has tended to use moral philosophy when political philosophy would be more appropriate, what sort of method could be used to demonstrate this? The claim is clearly an empirical one—bioethics only has a "problem" if we look at the bioethics literature and find that political philosophy is indeed missing. How could such a thing be accomplished in any kind of rigorous way?[2] But these sweeping claims also raise serious normative and philosophical issues. Who decides what the most important discipline is for addressing any particular question? Isn't the idea that political philosophy is the "best" tool for some job itself a normative claim? How would we even know if political philosophy were used *enough*? Wouldn't the answer to such a question depend, in part, on answering questions about which moral and political theory is the right one?

The book is in fact designed around these questions. To give a spoiler: there is no rigorous way to make the claim I am making. That is why I will have to combine broad characterization of the literature with specific, pointed examples, that I think are strong but are still, ultimately, only suggestive. Readers will have to judge for themselves whether the examples are compelling enough to demonstrate a problem with the field. Furthermore, there is no definitive way to explain the role that political philosophy *should* play in the bioethics literature without assuming a normative standpoint. That is why—after some broad observations of the field in chapters 1 and 2—I will stick to evaluating the bioethics literature from a specific normative standpoint, namely, a Kantian one. But the reasons for bringing Kant into this debate are, ultimately, related to showing the broader problem with the bioethics literature. Using moral instead of political theories for answering normative questions about health law and policy is a problem from many standpoints, although it is particularly problematic from a Kantian standpoint, as Kant himself made a great effort to demonstrate, I shall argue. But Kantian bioethicists have not generally considered the theoretical problems with trying to enforce Kantian morality; nor have they paid any attention to Kant's political philosophy, or any competing political philosophy; and what is more, they haven't been challenged to do so by their critics. This overall state of affairs is among the most damning evidence possible, I will argue that there is a problem with the field. If anyone should be employing political philosophy, and specifically a theory of government legitimacy, for practical problems it should be Kantian bioethicists. But instead of paying close attention to the conceptual issues with enforcing Kantian morality, or trying to apply the principles specifically developed by Kant for issues of law and policy, Kantian bioethicists have taken the same approach toward matters of law and policy that other bioethicists have: they justify laws and policies by appealing to principles and duties characteristic of moral philosophy, rather than by giving an account of the role and legitimate function of the government.

THE BOOK

The book will proceed in two very unequal parts. In the first and shorter part of the book (essentially chapters 1 and 2), I will make the case that political philosophy has been underrepresented in bioethics. In this part of the book the argument I make is mostly empirical and can be summarized by three major points. The first two occur in chapter 1. First, I argue that bioethics is, and always has been, oriented toward questions of law and policy—arguably the larger part of the discipline has been aimed at questions relating to law and policy, and has not been content with mere discussion of what behaviors are "moral" or "immoral." Even the principles most closely associated with bioethics were originally adopted in the context of pressing problems in health law and policy. My claim then is that bioethics has always been in practice a kind of applied political theorizing, since the questions bioethicists sought to answer were so often legal or regulatory ones. Even clinical bioethics depends in a very significant way on conclusions about the normative justifiability of laws and policies. Then I will discuss in a very abstract way the methods that would seem to be most appropriate to answering questions about the normative justification of laws and policies. What kinds of premises would be necessary to decide, for example, whether some action should be legally mandated, incentivized, or prohibited? This leads us to the second major point: premises about government are necessary for justifying any normative claim about health law or policy. Treating issues of law and policy as mere questions about the morality of the behaviors they regulate is problematic, because such an approach necessarily relies on premises about government that are rarely even articulated, let alone defended as part of a broader theoretical perspective.

The third major point in this first part of the book appears in chapter 2. Despite the field's aspiration to give arguments justifying health law and policy; and, despite the formal importance of normative theories about government to this project; political theory plays only a very small role in bioethics. The reasons for the absence of political philosophy in bioethics can be understood by studying the context in which the field emerged. Understanding that context sheds some light on why the major approaches present in the bioethics literature today have systematically marginalized theories of government and exposes some common but problematic assumptions these major approaches make about how law and policy should be justified. Political philosophy is nearly absent from major works on bioethics methodology, and the methods that these works have established has meant that it is also missing in most other areas of the field. We can see this by examining a variety of introductions to bioethics and general works on bioethics and law, for example. The argument is not that political philosophy is entirely absent from bioethics, but that it is severely underrepresented when considered in light of the political goals of the field and the wide (although by no means universal) enthusiasm the field shows for using philosophy as a method for justifying normative claims.

The second part of the book (chapters 3–8) will make a more sustained case for the inclusion of political philosophy in bioethics by using Kantian moral and political philosophy to give a detailed account of the problems with the dominant approach to normative justification of health law and policy, and the ways in which a political philosophy can solve them. This part of the book, with the exception of chapter 3, is mostly normative. In chapter 3, I survey a variety of ways that bioethicists have approached the question about whether markets in organs should be legally prohibited. I focus specifically on Kantian approaches to this question. This makes a comprehensive survey of the literature more feasible, but it also offers important insight about the way bioethicists approach questions of health law and policy. In that chapter I show how, despite a rich theoretical literature exploring multiple aspects of Kantian philosophy and applying it in diverse ways to the question of the legalization of organ markets, almost no attention has been given in that literature to basic questions about political philosophy, such as the conditions for legitimate laws, or the moral justification for the exercise of political power. This is perplexing because Kant himself devoted much attention to these issues in his political philosophy, developed in several of his works not often utilized in the bioethics literature. Instead, bioethicists have almost universally preferred to utilize Kant's moral philosophy to answer questions about the basic justifiability of laws prohibiting the sale of organs. In this way, they reflect the "moral philosophy approach" dominant in the bioethics literature, by which I mean that they determine the justifiability of laws and policies by using moral philosophy to determine whether the actions regulated are moral or immoral.

In chapter 4, I give a detailed account of the theoretical problems with this moral philosophy approach to issues of health law and policy. To do this, I give an account of the main problem associated with justifying specific health laws or policies (the problem of political legitimacy). I show why there is no easy way to solve the problem of legitimacy if we are limited to familiar moral principles described in Kantian moral philosophy. Although bioethicists in the literature on Kant and organ markets have thought that Kantian moral principles can explain either why we should or should not have legal prohibitions on organ sales, a careful study of Kant's moral philosophy shows that such uses Categorically misunderstand Kantian moral philosophy. The various versions of Kant's Categorical Imperative cannot easily justify any uses of political power, because for Kant moral duty is primarily about acting on the right reasons, and laws and policies have no way of causing us to do this. In fact, far from solving the problem of political legitimacy, Kant's Categorical Imperative actually presents three serious challenges for justifying political legitimacy, and so threatens to show that law and policy cannot be justified *at all*. The challenges presented by a careful reading of Kant's moral philosophy leave us in need of a dedicated account of the moral justification of exercise of political power—in other words, a normative political philosophy.

Fortunately, Kant provides such an account in his *Doctrine of Right*. In chapters 5 and 6 I develop an account of political legitimacy and authority along the lines of Kant's account in the *Doctrine of Right*, and argue that it solves the challenges that his familiar moral principles, taken by themselves, cannot. In chapter 5 I argue that Kant shows how the exercise of coercion is morally justified by the possibility of it being exercised in a manner consistent with the external freedom of everyone under universal law. Kant's account of the basic case of justified coercion helps solve some of the problems set up in chapter 4 but leaves others outstanding. In chapter 6, I argue that Kant provides the resources for answering these remaining challenges in his accounts of private and public right and I show how he does so. Notably, I also argue here that Kant's political philosophy is actually necessary for plausibly applying his moral philosophy to many *moral*, rather than political, questions. A theory of political rights of the kind Kant provides turns out to be a necessary precursor to answering basic questions about whether actions use persons as a mere means, on my account.

In chapters 7 and 8, I explore some ways in which political philosophy—in this case, the Kantian one I developed in chapters 5 and 6—might change the bioethics debate surrounding two significant legal issues in bioethics. These chapters illustrate some ways that significant issues and questions have been overlooked in the bioethics literature because it has utilized methods of moral philosophy, rather than more appropriate methods characteristic of political philosophy. These chapters are important for understanding the fundamental rethinking of various bioethics issues that normative political philosophy can offer us.

In chapter 7, I rethink the contribution Kant makes to questions about the legal permissibility of markets in organs. While chapter 3 shows how Kant is usually interpreted as supporting laws prohibiting the sale of kidneys, his basic political principles suggest that governments actually lack the authority to legally prohibit such sales. This is true even though such sales are deeply immoral, on his view. However, Kant's theory also provides reasons for thinking that the state cannot legitimately enforce contracts for kidney sales. I argue, then, that the considered Kantian position on such markets is that they must be legally permitted, although contracts for kidneys are unenforceable. The stark contrast between "Kantian" accounts based on his moral views, and the most defensible position based on his political ones, illustrates the importance of political philosophy for justifying law and policy. Laws that seem easily justified by their role in enforcing "morality" may turn out to be deeply unjustifiable when considered more carefully in light of the principles defining and limiting the legitimate exercise of political power.

In chapter 8 I rethink the basis of informed consent laws. Bioethicists have typically utilized the moral philosophy approach here as they have elsewhere, thinking that laws requiring informed consent must be justified on the basis of our general moral rights. But they have failed to justify informed consent laws, I argue, because they have not been able to explain why general pre-political rights to consent entail that physicians (alone among parties seeking to obtain consent) have special duties to inform patients about the risks and benefits of treatment. The Kantian political approach is different, because it starts with the presupposition that our prepolitical moral rights are indeterminate. So although patients have a basic moral right to consent, nothing specific follows from this about how much information physicians must give patients in order to obtain a valid consent. Physicians consequently have no specific prepolitical duties to inform patients prior to treating them. However, Kant understands this condition of indeterminate prepolitical rights and duties as deeply morally problematic, and it forms the basis of his account of government authority. The government exists in part to solve the problem of indeterminacy and give content to our prepolitical moral rights, as part of its general mandate to make us equal under law. Because the government has authority to determine the specific contours of, for example, the physician's duties when obtaining consent, it can endow physicians with both a moral and legal duty to inform patients about the benefits and risks of treatment as a condition for obtaining a valid consent. In this case, political philosophy is not only necessary for determining the nature of our political rights and obligations, but also for giving shape and content to our moral duties.

THEORY AND BIOETHICS: A FEW CONCERNS

As I've said, the primary purpose of this book is to argue for reconsidering the importance of political philosophy or political theory to bioethics. I argue that bioethics should use principles explaining the legitimacy of governmental actions when justifying laws or policies. However, some readers may be skeptical about the importance of theory *in general* (moral or political) for bioethics. If theory in general is not a legitimate or important way of treating bioethics issues, then it may seem misguided to suggest that political philosophy has an important role to play in the justification of law and policy. Other readers may think theory is important, but question the relevance of specific kinds of theories, such as the kind of Kantian theory I've indicated will be employed in this book.

Critics have had a variety of motivations and have questioned the use of theory in bioethics in different ways. Some writers—such as casuists—have been skeptical about the use of theory in moral reasoning altogether.[3] Obviously, if theory should not play a significant role in moral reasoning, then arguments about "what kind" of theory we should employ in bioethics will lose much of their interest. In this book, I make the modest assumption that moral and political theorizing is sometimes valuable for bioethical reasoning.

Even granting this modest claim, some may object that theory is nevertheless a liability in certain contexts. For example, Will Kymlicka argues against the use of theory on governmental commissions, in part because there is limited time in this context to engage in extensive theorizing.[4] John Arras, similarly, argues against the use of theory in the public policy context, because the more "theoretical" the work is, the less likely that it can be understood by the general population, and so the less likely that it can be endorsed in a meaningful way by the electorate from which laws get their authority in a democratic society.[5]

The argument in this book, however, is not for the use of theory in any particular context. The argument is instead a qualitative one: it is about the kind of theory that should be employed when we engage in theory, not an account about when we should engage in it. If there are certain contexts where overt theory is not appropriate—as there likely are—then political philosophy should not be used in those contexts, but neither should moral theory. The argument here is best understood in a hypothetical sense: if theory is ever justified in bioethics reasoning about law and policy, then it is political rather than moral theorizing that deserves pride of place. The argument in chapter 1, that normative claims about laws and policies presumably must rely on some account about what governments should generally do, should be taken in this way. It may not always be appropriate for bioethicists to explain the more general premises about morality or political legitimacy that lead to their conclusions about law and policy; but if they do, it is indefensible to explain only the relevant moral premises, and not the (even more) relevant political ones.

KANTIAN THEORY

A different set of concerns has been leveled not at the context of theoretical work, but instead at the kinds of theories employed. Specifically, some have argued against the use of "high moral theory," particularly theories of the kind traditionally studied in normative ethics, such as Kantian or utilitarian theories.[6] Various concerns about these theories are raised, including their "architectonic" nature (meaning that they usually depend on one or a few foundational principles—which, if wrong, would seem to invalidate the whole theory), and the background pluralism that makes appeal to such theories controversial, or even morally objectionable. In some ways, it is possible to read the whole field of bioethics as a response to the problem of pluralism about morality and the necessity of finding commonly acceptable solutions to moral problems. I explore this reading of the field in chapter 2.

From this perspective, it may seem like appeals to Kantian moral or political philosophy rest on a very significant misunderstanding of bioethics and its tasks in the real world. On this view, bioethics exists to present commonly acceptable answers to our public problems, not to further divide us by appealing to controversial or outdated theories.

However, part of the argument of this book is that we have lost something in the move away from the use of "high" moral and political theory. Specifically, I argue in chapter 2 that bioethics moved toward mid-level principles—such as, for example, Beauchamp and Childress's four principles of biomedical ethics—as a practical way of avoiding some of the controversy that threatened to undermine bioethics deliberation in the pluralistic context of health care. However, the move to mid-level principles unwittingly focused attention on what I call "primary moral duties," that is, moral duties ordinary persons have toward one another. Because of the focus on these primary moral duties, bioethicists have predominantly considered issues of law and policy through that lens: not as questions about the duties and rights of governments, but instead as questions about the duties of professionals (or in some cases, citizens or patients). Conclusions about these are then translated directly into law or policy.

The problems with this approach are best seen by taking a step back and considering, abstractly, whether an account of these primary moral duties is sufficient for justifying either law or policy. I argue that it is not, but the argument is necessarily theoretical. For example, in order to consider whether showing that something is immoral is enough to show that it should also be illegal, we have to consider what it means for something to be "immoral" in the first place. Kantian theory is employed in part because it makes a commitment about major concepts explored here, such as "morality," "coercion," "legitimacy," and more.

I caution readers against what would, in my view, be a serious misreading of this book. Some readers may be tempted to read this as merely a "Kantian political account" of bioethics. This book does provide the outlines of such an approach, but I will spend relatively little time defending Kant's particular political philosophy against competing political approaches (although, I do provide an extensive argument about why Kant's political philosophy is preferable to his moral philosophy when addressing issues of law and policy). The main argument of the book is that bioethics should use political philosophy when justifying health law and policy, and I employ Kant's moral and political theory as a way of showing what is at stake and why it is important. Kant is particularly helpful for this project because he provides a detailed and thorough account about the principled distinctions between moral obligation and political legitimacy. Much of the potential audience for this book does, I suspect, self-consciously reject Kantian moral theory for one reason or other. As we will discuss in some detail (especially in chapter 5), the main principles of Kantian political theory are not directly dependent on his moral principles, even though they are compatible with them. So I encourage readers to approach Kant's political theory with an open mind, even if they reject Kant's moral theory. But even if readers have reasons for rejecting both his moral and political theory, I think this book still has something to offer them: it is a book about the importance of normative political philosophy, and not just a Kantian political bioethics.

Because the main purpose of the book is to reflect on the relationship between morality and law, and to consider the reasons why political theory is more suited to addressing health law and policy problems than moral theory, it is important to regard the normative policy conclusions of chapters 7 and 8 somewhat tentatively. In both chapters, I draw normative conclusions about policy on the basis of Kantian arguments about the source and nature of government legitimacy and authority. I believe that these conclusions are relatively better justified than other positions on these issues in the extant literature. However, part of the reason why Kant's theory is relatively successful here compared to the existing bioethics literature is that few authors in bioethics are even addressing the relevant questions in these applied cases—namely, questions about the source, nature, and limitations of the state's legitimacy and authority. If we had a more robust literature beginning with these questions rather than questions about our moral duties, then Kantian political philosophy could be put into fruitful exchange with other views about government legitimacy and authority, and we might find (methodologically appropriate) reasons for thinking that the Kantian positions I develop are wrong. If there ever comes a day when the bioethics literature engages more extensively with these issues from competing views about the legitimacy and authority of the government, then perhaps there will be occasion to revisit the normative conclusions of these chapters.

NOTES

1. By "moral philosophy" from here forward, I mean the branch of philosophy that develops theories that are meant to assess our most basic duties toward each other. By "political philosophy," I understand theories specifically designed to address questions about what makes government "just or legitimate or good" (see the discussion in chapter 1). On some accounts—including perhaps the Kantian one, as I discuss in chapter 5—political philosophy should be understood as a branch of moral philosophy. Even so, in this book I argue that the problems raised in attempting to justify governments and their laws go well beyond the more basic ones about our duties to each other that are the bread and butter of moral philosophy. As such they require additional explanation about concepts such as legitimacy and authority, even if political philosophy is ultimately best understood as a branch of moral philosophy broadly construed. This distinction between moral and political philosophy also underlies Kant's approach. In some works, such as the *Groundwork*, the *Critique of Practical Reason*, and the *Doctrine of Virtue*, Kant is most concerned with explaining our basic duties to one another. In others—most significantly, the *Doctrine of Right*, but also in his occasional works, such as "Theory and Practice," and "Towards Perpetual Peace"—Kant discusses issues related to government legitimacy and authority.

2. For a discussion of the value but also limitations of this kind of work, see Rosalind McDougall, "Systematic Reviews in Bioethics: Types, Challenges, and Value," *The Journal of Medicine and Philosophy* 39, no. 1 (2014).

3. Albert R. Jonsen, *The Birth of Bioethics* (New York: Oxford University Press, 1998), 333.

4. Will Kymlicka, "Moral Philosophy and Public Policy: The Case of New Reproductive Technologies," in *Philosophical Perspectives on Bioethics*, ed. L W Sumner and Joseph M Boyle (Toronto: University of Toronto Press, 1996).

5. John Arras, "Theory and Bioethics," in *The Stanford Encyclopedia of Philosophy*, ed. Edward N. Zalta (2020). https://plato.stanford.edu/archives/fall2020/entries/theory-bioethics/.

6. John Arras, "Theory and Bioethics," in *The Stanford Encyclopedia of Philosophy*, ed. Edward N. Zalta (2020).

Chapter 1

The Political Tasks of Bioethics

LAW AND POLICY IN BIOETHICS

A fifty-nine-year-old female with past history of congestive heart failure and atrial fibrillation arrives at the local emergency room after being found unresponsive at her home. In the ambulance, medics determine she has a Glasgow Coma Score of 3; she cannot breathe on her own, so medics intubate her. Upon arriving at the hospital, her CT scan reveals an ischemic middle cerebral artery stroke with hemorrhagic transformation. She is stabilized and admitted to the Intensive Care Unit.[1]

The patient has a living will stating that she does not wish to be maintained on a ventilator unless her recovery is likely and does not wish to be resuscitated while ventilator dependent. It also records her intention to donate her organs after death.

After several days, the patient has shown no improvement. The doctors explain to the family that she will not regain consciousness, and that they plan to remove the ventilator according to the instructions in her living will. The family objects because they think this will "kill" the patient. The physicians explain that they are legally required to follow the patient's directives, however, and that removing care is usually considered allowing the patient to die, rather than "killing" the patient.

The doctors further tell the family that the patient has authorized an anatomical gift by registering as an organ donor, and that they have planned an organ procurement operation after the patient dies. The family objects again because they do not like the idea of surgery after the patient's death. The doctors tell the family that the patient has a right to authorize this, and it is not their decision.

They ask the family if they would like to visit a final time. They may be present in the operating room following withdrawal of the ventilator until the patient's heart stops beating, but they will need to leave immediately afterward, so that the organ procurement team can begin their work. The family agrees to this plan after some discussion with the health care team.

At the appointed time, the family says goodbye to the patient in the operating room where the organs will be removed. The health care team removes the ventilator and the patient's heart stops beating. The family is escorted from the operating room. Exactly two minutes after the cessation of circulation, the procurement team goes to work removing two kidneys and a liver from the patient to be transplanted into someone else.

The Law in Clinical Medicine

Even though this story contains no police, judges, or lawmakers, laws and policies[2] circumscribe almost every decision in this story. These laws and policies have been the subject of extensive bioethics debate over the years, and some of them continue to be debated. Bioethicists have made important contributions to the development of these laws and policies. In many cases, we can trace a line between the laws that determine what happens in cases like these and specific reports or arguments given by ethicists, often in the context of their work for government commissions.

For example, the idea that patients rather than families or physicians decide about health care is one that has long held sway in American law.[3] However, the idea that patients have a right to refuse even life-sustaining care is more recent. This position was promoted in a report by a presidential commission entitled *Deciding to Forego Life-Sustaining Treatments*.[4] The Commission contained bioethicists and also relied on reports written by external bioethicists for reaching this conclusion.[5]

The right of the patient to refuse treatment in this case also raises the question about whether withdrawing treatment effectively *kills* the patient. It is one thing to omit implementing a life-sustaining treatment, but to many people (including the family in this case) *withdrawing* life-sustaining treatment does not seem like letting a patient die so much as actively killing her. If it did count as killing, then it would constitute euthanasia, which remains illegal in all states in the United States. But in *Deciding to Forego*, bioethicists argued that there is no morally significant difference between withholding and withdrawing treatment.[6] The Commission decided not to get involved in the terminological debate about what constitutes "killing," but argued instead that withdrawing life-sustaining treatment at the request of a competent patient is morally identical to withholding treatment at the request of a competent patient. Since physicians were already comfortable with withholding treatment, this effectively eased concerns about whether withdrawing life-sustaining treatment is "killing."

Beyond decisions about health care, a patient's authority to determine the fate of his or her organs after death is by no means obvious. While people generally have authority to determine the fate of their belongings through a legally binding will, the extension of wills to health care decisions—and eventually to the disposition of the patient's body parts after death—was an important one. The Uniform Anatomical Gift Act (UAGA) authorizes procurement of organs with a patient authorization, even when a family objects.[7]

Before taking the patient's organs, however, and in order to avoid charges of battery or even murder, physicians must determine that the patient is already dead. This is sometimes called the "dead donor rule." Organs cannot be utilized if they have been without oxygen for more than a few minutes. One of the reasons to define death clearly is to make it possible to procure organs as early as possible and so to minimize the time that an organ is at body temperature after its blood supply has been cut off. In the report *Defining Death*, bioethicists contributed to a proposed uniform definition of death that helped to clarify when organs could be harvested. The report defined death as either cessation of all brain activity (whole brain death) or irreversible cessation of respiratory and circulatory function.[8] This recommendation was soon incorporated into state laws as part of the Uniform Determination of Death Act (UDDA).[9] Cessation of circulation is usually understood as *irreversible* after at least two minutes have elapsed, because there is little evidence of spontaneous autoresuscitation after that point.

Although controlled donations after circulatory death (DCD)—that is, donations that follow a planned removal of life-sustaining care, in the absence of brain death, as this one is—account for only a small percentage of donations in the United States, the elaboration of a procedure for making such donations was necessitated in part by the very long waiting list for organs in the United States. That is, controlled DCD is one means of increasing the organ supply for those who badly need organs and may die without them. The existence of a long waiting list for access to organs is, arguably, created in part by the legal prohibition of other means of organ distribution—such as a market in kidneys[10]—which was accomplished by the National Organ Transplant Act of 1984 (NOTA). The ethical principles thought to justify this policy approach are elaborated by the Organ Procurement and Transplantation Network (OPTN), a body created under NOTA and given authority to regulate organ distribution in the United States. OPTN understands its approach to organ distribution as undergirded by the ethical principles developed in the *Belmont Report*,[11] a report developed by the first national bioethics commission in the United States, drafted by and in consultation with a number of bioethicists.

Asking the Right Questions about Law and Policy

One set of questions we can ask when evaluating the laws governing cases like these is whether the actions they require are ethical. This was in fact the main kind of question that was asked by bioethicists who made the policy recommendations governing these cases. These questions include: what sort of cognitive capacities make a patient's decision about health care worth respecting? What moral values are at risk if physicians or families, rather than patients themselves, make decisions about health care? Is there a moral difference between withholding and withdrawing care? Is there a moral difference between killing and letting die? Is a patient who has ceased breathing already dead, such that it is not possible that removing vital organs from such patients *kills* them? Would it be morally wrong to kill a patient who consents, in any case? Is it ever morally permissible to take a vital organ from one patient and put it in the body of another patient, even after death? These are all important questions, and they have been treated extensively by bioethicists, both in their work for government reports and, of course, extensively in the literature they have produced dealing with these issues.

Whatever we might think about the answers to these various ethical questions, it is critical to realize that these questions are not the most important questions to ask about the laws and policies governing a case like this one. The ethical questions are about the moral qualities of the actions that are regulated. But there is also a group of second-order questions that must be asked about the actions of those who make, interpret, and enforce laws and policies regulating health care. These activities are conceptually distinct from the activities of those who give or receive care, and they raise a distinct set of moral questions. What justifies the criminalization of seemingly self-regarding actions, such as buying or selling organs, or use of medical-grade drugs for recreation? What justifies the state's extensive efforts to control the distribution of, and access to, health care resources? What justifies the legal regulation of the practice of medicine in general? For example, governments restrict the practice of medicine to those it deems qualified medical practitioners and criminalizes practicing law without a license. What gives the government authority to restrict medicine in this way? Governments further determine much of the content of the practice of medicine: deciding, for example, that administering drugs for pain is medicine, but administering drugs for the purpose of suicide is not. But they also decide on what may otherwise seem like medical issues: when is a patient alive, and when dead? What is a disease, and who decides?

These questions are often answered by appealing directly to Constitutional or other legal sources. But they can also be considered as moral questions: not questions about what the government has the *legal* authority to do, but instead about what it has *moral* authority to do, or what it should do. These questions, while vital for making any kind of normative recommendation for health law or policy, have rarely been significant parts of deliberation leading up to the passage of the laws that have so much influence in the practice of medicine.

Justifying Law and Policy

When thinking about laws and policies, then, we need to ask not only "first-order" questions about the ethics of the practices that are regulated, but also "second-order" questions: questions about what justifies the laws and policies that regulate, prohibit, mandate, incentivize, and in other ways affect the relationships and activities in health care.

This is a book about the tools required for justifying law and policy. In this book, I will offer an answer to the question about how law and policy can be justified. However, offering that answer is not the main purpose of this book. Instead, the purpose is to offer an extended argument that bioethics does not, but should, address questions about the purpose and role of the government when evaluating laws and policies. I will argue, in short, that what bioethics needs is political philosophy, particularly the kind that addresses the source of the government's legitimacy.

Before giving an account about how this approach might work, however, I want to make an initial case for the necessity of political philosophy in bioethics. In this chapter, we will give summary consideration to the importance of political philosophy for bioethics. In the following part of this chapter (Law and Policy in Bioethics) I will argue that one of the crucial tasks of the field is, and always has been, giving normative evaluation of law and policy. That this has always been considered a task of bioethics is evident from the attempts of bioethicists to give policy advice even before the "discipline" of bioethics was born. I will argue that interest in justifying changes to law and policy is considerably more pervasive in the field than might initially be apparent. The task of bioethics to give normative evaluation to law and policy does not end with policy advice, however. This is because even clinical bioethics work often implicitly depends on a normative evaluation of the laws and policies regulating clinical practice. Consequently, even bioethicists whose work seems far removed from the work of policy advocates or government commissions must necessarily consider the moral justifiability of various laws and policies governing the practice of clinical ethics.

After arguing for the overall importance of normative evaluation of law and policy for bioethics, in the final part of this chapter (How to Justify Law and Policy) I will make a preliminary argument for why bioethics needs political philosophy to accomplish this task. I will argue that normative evaluation of laws and policies is incomplete without political philosophy.

In chapter 2, I will assess the extent to which bioethics has, and makes use of, the tools appropriate for justifying law and policy. I will argue that the basic tools much of the field uses to approach questions about law and policy—moral principles and theories—are not sufficient for this task. Certain basic features of these theories and principles make them conceptually inadequate for addressing these problems. Together, these arguments in chapters 1 and 2 make a preliminary case that bioethics needs, but does not have, adequate tools for the normative tasks associated with justifying health law and policy and clears the ground for the more detailed discussion in the remainder of the book.

LAW AND POLICY IN BIOETHICS

Public Policy Advice

Political Aims from the Beginning

Bioethicists' interest in health law and policy can be traced all the way back to the beginning of the field. By the time that the term "bioethics" was coined—apparently independently, by Van Rensselaer Potter (in a 1970 article[12]) and Sargent Shriver (in discussions with Andre Hellegers in 1970)[13]—the Hastings Center had already been formed for the purpose of studying the ethics of the "life sciences." The inception of the Hastings Center in 1969[14] marked a milestone in the development of bioethics as a field because it was the first institution dedicated to evaluating the ethics of medicine and life sciences from an external perspective—that is, from outside of the professions being evaluated. The trends that made social investigation of the practices of medicine and life sciences seem necessary, as Albert Jonsen notes in a history of bioethics, had been widely noticed: they included the increasing prominence of health care research; the discovery of DNA, which suggested the prospect of genetic manipulation; the development of artificial ventilation; the first heart transplant; and the development of the "external kidney," or hemodialysis.[15] These developments gave medicine a level of control over birth, life, and death that was unprecedented. They also raised a host of seemingly novel questions about the ethical use of these technologies, as well as complicated questions about how new technologies should be funded and distributed. Within just a few years after the founding of the Hastings Center, bioethics was recognized as a "discipline" by the Library of Congress,[16] and a variety of other institutions, programs, and initiatives dedicated to studying bioethics had formed, including the Kennedy Institute of Ethics, the Society for Health and Human Values, and the first national commission on bioethics.

Interest in law and policy was pervasive among these early groups. Daniel Callahan, the founder (along with Willard Gaylin) of the Hastings Center, published a book entitled *Abortion: Law, Choice and Morality* the year after the center was founded.[17] The inaugural annual meeting at the Hastings Center in 1971 was entitled, "Heart Transplants and Public Policy."[18] Albert Jonsen recounts being invited to the Center for monthly meetings on ethics and public policy.[19]

Similar political interests were present from the beginning at the nascent Kennedy Institute of Ethics at Georgetown University, formed in 1971. Senator Kennedy, speaking at the opening of the Kennedy Institute, spoke of the "future importance of bioethics for the formation of public policy."[20] The first set of scholars at the Institute wrote books with titles such as *Politics, Medicine and Christian Ethics: A Dialogue with Paul Ramsey*, and "Social Justice and Equal Access to Health Care."[21] Bioethicists' interest in evaluating and proposing law and policy was present in the field from its beginning.

Formal Involvement in Law and Policy

Bioethics had barely begun when bioethicists began playing a more formal role in setting law and policy. The clearest example of this can be seen in the role that bioethicists played as members of, and consultants for, national bioethics commissions.

The first of these commissions was called by Congress in 1973. The National Commission for the Protection of Human Subjects of Biomedical and Behavioral Research (informally, the Belmont Commission) was asked by Congress to perform several tasks, but its general mandate was to identify basic ethical principles for the use of human subjects in research. This was a remarkable request: as Jonsen comments, "No legislation had ever before charged a government body 'to identify basic ethical principles' as did Public Law 93–348."[22]

The Commission's report identifying these ethical principles—the *Belmont Report*[23]—redacted the work of multiple professional moral philosophers and theologians commissioned to write essays on pertinent topics. It identified three moral "principles," general enough to be considered common to our culture but also specific enough to provide some normative content: the principles of respect for persons, beneficence, and justice. The *Report* was incorporated in its entirety into the *Federal Register* (the official journal of the proceedings of federal government),[24] and currently forms the backbone for United States federal regulation of human subjects research in the Common Rule (45 CFR §46).

The Common Rule is a legal policy for health care only in the sense that it regulates the uses of federal research funds. Private research performed by entities not receiving federal dollars are not bound by the principles established by the *Belmont Report*, or its associated rules. Although the Rule ostensibly governs the use of federal research funds, in fact its influence is far more pervasive than this suggests. This is so in a formal sense because the Rule requires the establishment of Institutional Review Boards (IRBs) at institutions that receive federal funding. Since nearly all universities in the United States and many corporations receive or aspire to receive such funding, this stipulation effectively governs most institutions conducting research on human subjects in the United States, and many abroad.

But the *Report* also created a precedent that paved the way for even more extensive formal involvement of bioethics in law and policy. Part of this "precedent-setting" effect was due to the overall success of the Commission. The Commission performed an important service by clarifying a relatively simple set of guidelines that could prevent research abuse. Moreover, the Commission's overall methodology—requiring the specification of several mid-level that were more general than the issues to which they were applied, but less general than traditional theories of normative ethics—was broadly acceptable in a pluralistic secular context, and so could serve as the theoretical foundation for the activities of future committees. We will discuss the advantages and implications of this theoretical approach in more detail in chapter 2.

For these and probably other reasons, a continuing role for national bioethics commissions, utilizing a set of abstract and secular principles to make recommendations for law and policy, seemed attractive. President Jimmy Carter appointed his own national commission, the President's Commission, almost immediately after the dissolution of the Belmont Commission. This Commission wrote reports on a wide variety of topics relating to law and policy, such as the legal permissibility of withholding or withdrawing life-sustaining care, the legal definition of death, the laws and policies governing informed consent, and the implementation of a legal right to health care. Bioethicists often served directly on this and other commissions, and bioethicists who were not commission members often played a substantial role in writing background papers whose arguments and conclusions found their way into the reports issued by the Commission. Even when the recommendations of these commissions were about the "ethics" of various issues, they generally included sections on recommendations for public policy in their reports.

In many cases these reports had a discernible impact on public policy. For example, Gray found in 1993 that the report *Deciding to Forego Life-Sustaining Treatment* had already been cited three times in Supreme

Court rulings and had appeared in numerous other "prominent" court cases as well.[25] The report *Defining Death* had even greater impact on public policy, because it gave formal input in the development of Uniform Determination of Death Act, a uniform legal standard that was quickly adopted by nearly all U.S. states.

Because the reports themselves are not (excepting the *Belmont Report*) actual public policy, it is sometimes difficult to determine the precise amount of influence these reports have on laws. For example, Baruch Brody argues that the report *Deciding to Forego Life-Sustaining Treatment*, while broadly credited with altering policy, in fact merely represented an emerging consensus about many of the issues it addresses, and so was not directly responsible for the changes.[26] The laws and policies developed after these reports are likely influenced to varying degrees by the reports, and there is often no way of determining the precise amount of influence of any one report. Nevertheless, the process by which the reports are produced, their stated aims, and the references to them in the surrounding literature provide abundant evidence of the public policy orientation of these commissions and the bioethics arguments and theories they rely on.

The tradition of inviting academics and especially moral philosophers to comment on the morality of various public policy and regulatory issues has, since these early days, become somewhat institutionalized. About ten national bioethics commissions have since been convened, usually either by Congress or by executive order.[27] President Obama, for example, began appointments for his commission a few months after inauguration.[28] Bioethicists have consistently called for new bioethics commissions during the recent Trump and Biden presidencies, which further demonstrates the importance of such bodies to the field.[29]

Informal Involvement in Law and Policy

Interest in affecting law and public policy through venues such as national commissions (as well as many other less visible venues, such as state commissions and legally protected professional associations) has played an important role in shaping the whole field, even when there is no formal connection to law or policy.

In a sociological history, John Evans traces the impact of the Belmont Commission and its associated principles on public bioethics debate surrounding human genetic engineering in the United States.[30] Evans explains that the debate on human genetic engineering, prior to Belmont, had been wide-ranging, had been conducted most often by theologians, and that it had relied on ultimate values. Evans argues that this approach was quickly eclipsed in the literature surrounding this issue after the advent of the principles pioneered by the Belmont Commission, which were relatively "thin" and concerned mostly with determining whether actions were efficient at achieving given values. Applying these principles required no theological training and invoked no ultimate values.

Evans illustrates the process by which the principles of Belmont came to replace earlier methods in the academic literature by showing the ripple effects of a government commission on human genetic engineering (HGE) on the academic literature surrounding that topic. According to Evans, soon after the establishment of the Human Gene Therapy Subcommittee of the Recombinant DNA Advisory Commission (RAC) in the 1980s (hereafter, the Subcommittee), government advisory commissions—rather than, for example, other scholars or the public—became "the consumer and target of ethical arguments about [human genetic engineering]."[31] As Evans states, if authors on this topic wanted to have any influence on the HGE debate, they had to write in a way that was "suited" to the Subcommittee.[32] The Subcommittee had accepted the Belmont principles (respect for persons, beneficence, and justice) as the acceptable methodology for approaching questions about HGE. Consequently, the literature on this topic quickly changed so as to be characterized by discussion of these principles and their implications for HGE, effectively driving out the approaches utilized by theologians before them. Evans considers the various contributions to the literature on germline HGE during the period when the Subcommittee was working on these issues. According to Evans, the majority of influential authors writing on this topic during that period were formally tied to the government (they were government ethicists, commission chairs, or government bodies themselves). The dominance of government-affiliated authors writing on the topic virtually assured that the rest of the field would have to pay heed to the values, goals, and methods of those influential authors. And indeed they did—as Evans notes, of the four most influential articles on HGE not written by these government authors during this period, three mention in the first paragraph that the Subcommittee is the target of their ethical advice.[33] In sum, Evans argues that formal government involvement in the ethics of HGE quickly changed the scholarly literature surrounding the issue because bioethicists had to adopt the language and methods acceptable to the government commission if their work was to have any influence on law or policy.

By establishing the form of argument developed at Belmont as the acceptable approach to a series of consecutive issues treated by government commissions, "the form of argument itself came to be reified as normative for all ethical questions"[34] This form of argument gradually came to characterize the whole bioethics literature, not just the part directly addressing issues of law and policy. Because the field attached so much importance to affecting laws and policies, they had to adopt the methodology regnant in government bodies charged with considering questions about law and policy. The method that they ultimately adopted en route to their policy and law goals—the principles characteristic of Belmont and (as we shall later see) the related principlism of the important authors Beauchamp and Childress—is itself evidence of the law and policy aspirations of the field, even when law and policy are not directly under consideration.

Considering the Subject Matter of Bioethics

A less-historical way of determining the importance of law and policy aims to bioethics is by surveying the content of bioethics textbooks, particularly anthologies. Although bioethics textbooks are typically marketed toward undergraduate students, rather than government commissions or policy makers, their contents nevertheless can help us appreciate the extent to which the content of bioethics is focused on law and policy. Consider the major topic headings from the table of contents of one widely used anthology of bioethics literature, *Ethical Issues in Modern Medicine*.[35]

1.1 Autonomy, paternalism and medical models
1.2 Informed consent
1.3 Conflicting professional roles and responsibilities
2.1 Justice and health care
2.2 Methods and strategies for rationing health care
2.3 Equality and the ends of medicine
3.1 The definition of death
3.2 Decisional capacity and the right to refuse treatment
3.3 Advance directives
3.4 Choosing for others
3.5 Euthanasia and physician-assisted suicide
4.1 The morality of abortion
4.2 Carrier screening, prenatal testing, and reproductive decisions
4.3 Mapping the human genome
4.4 Assisted reproductive technologies
4.5 Human cloning and stem cell research
5.1 Born in scandal: The origins of U.S. research ethics
5.2 The ethics of randomized clinical trials
5.3 Ethical issues in international research
5.4 Research on children and other 'vulnerable' populations

A quick survey of the articles contained under each of the listed headings shows the following. Twelve out of the twenty sections contain articles that are either extracted directly from political documents (such as written opinions from court cases, government commission reports, or international laws) or whose titles directly reference some political document. Of the remaining eight that do not contain such articles, four are about issues that have been heavily legislated and subjected to political debate (2.2 and 2.3 about health care rationing, 4.1 about abortion, and 4.4 about assisted reproductive technologies). Many of the articles in the remaining four sections make major policy recommendations although they do not make this apparent in their titles (for example, see Glantz et al., suggesting new regulations governing international researchers and their funders in section 5.3;[36] or Emanuel and Emanuel, suggesting the "deliberative model" for informed consent laws in section 1.2;[37] etc.). Other major anthologies are organized in a similar way, and a brief review of their contents yields much the same result.[38]

Those familiar with the debates on each of these issues will know that there is not a single issue in the table of contents above that does not have significant policy-related aspects that are widely understood in the field. In many cases, we know this because the issues at stake in the scholarly literature are the laws themselves, and authors take specific laws as the items of their focus. For example, much of the literature about the just distribution of health and health care aims to propose a rationale for reforming laws and policies governing the distribution of health care.

In other cases, authors may omit to mention their views about policy issues, precisely because they think they are too obvious to mention. For example, much of the literature on physician-assisted suicide and euthanasia fits this description. Discussions of physician-assisted suicide (PAS) and euthanasia have had a place in bioethics curricula and textbooks since nearly the beginning of the field. Much of the debate centers around the "ethics" or "morality" of these activities. As interesting as the question about the ethics of these activities is, arguably the "ethics" of either has been (and continues to be) a moot point in most jurisdictions *unless* one is also interested in the public policy implications of the debate. This is straightforwardly because both remain illegal in most jurisdictions and are associated with steep legal penalties. Operating on the assumption that an immoral killing should be criminalized, bioethicists can seemingly stick to a question about the ethics of euthanasia or PAS while implicitly assessing the laws or policies that prohibit it. To demonstrate that either PAS or euthanasia or both are, at least in some cases, "ethical," is to go a long way in resolving the associated legal problems.[39] This is not to say, of course, that discussing ethical questions about PAS and euthanasia might not be interesting in its own right, as a purely intellectual endeavor. But the prominence of the topic is difficult to understand except in light of the surrounding legal and policy battles. Other debates, such as those over the ethics of embryonic stem cell research and abortion, are (at least in the United States) much the same. Because the legal implications are widely agreed to be "obvious," the debate about the law can proceed almost entirely without even mentioning the associated laws. The best way of understanding whether an article has legal ambitions, in such cases, is by asking whether the conclusions of the ethical argument it presents would (if successful) have legal implications obvious to most people.

In other cases background beliefs or views about the role or purpose of law can make an issue implicitly legal when it otherwise might not be. For example, Beauchamp and Faden write about "two senses" of informed consent: one is the moral ideal of an autonomous authorization and the other is the policies and institutional structures surrounding the practice of informed consent. According to them, the moral ideal of autonomous authorization ought to serve as the "benchmark" for policies governing informed consent.[40] Given this background belief, any discussion about ideal consent interactions will necessarily have legal implications, because the purpose of laws is to uphold an ethical ideal.

Clinical Ethics Advice

This is not to say that all bioethics literature is primarily political in its intent. Ezekiel Emanuel would seem to go too far when he says that bioethics is a "subfield of political philosophy."[41] Presumably, there are issues of bioethics that neither depend on nor immediately implicate any policy or political stance.

However, as medicine becomes an increasingly dominant sector of the economy and the regulations surrounding it continue to grow, it becomes increasingly difficult to think of any examples of completely apolitical issues. The political aspect of the field is hard to avoid, even in discussions that appear to be merely about clinical ethics.

Giving clinical ethics advice is necessarily a partly political task because so much of clinical practice is regulated by law and policy. We saw this at the beginning of the chapter: laws and policies regulate many aspects of clinical practice, such as who can make their own decisions, when a patient's decision must be considered legally binding, the circumstances under which physicians' actions are considered causal for the patient's condition, what counts as death, and when physicians may remove organs from one patient and place them in another.

There are different understandings of the role of the clinical ethicist, but no matter how this role is conceived, the clinical ethicist seemingly must have some idea about the significance of law and policy for determining what counts as "ethical" practice in the clinic.

For example, on one view the clinical ethicist gives substantive moral advice to those with whom they consult.[42] But if clinical ethicists are to give substantive moral advice about what is ethical, they must take a position on the laws that seek to constrain decision making in clinical practice. They must take into consideration, for example, whether there is a duty to obey relevant laws or not, before it is possible for them to advise others on what are the "ethical" decisions to make within such a heavily regulated context. For example, imagine a patient in great pain and with a terminal illness who requests a drug for the purpose of suicide, in a jurisdiction where physician-assisted suicide is illegal. Before recommending that the physician should dispense the drug, an ethicist will have to consider whether it is possible that the law can create an ethical obligation for the physician, even if none would exist absent that law. It is possible, in other words, that laws can create moral duties for physicians where those would not otherwise exist. It is impossible to give all-things-considered ethical advice to proceed, in such a situation without some consideration about whether law can create such duties, and whether this particular law does.

Or suppose that most clinical ethicists would *not* recommend assisting in suicide in this case, as is perhaps more likely. They cannot make such a recommendation on the basis of the laws if they do not know whether the laws create moral obligations for physicians. If they recommend against assisting merely because assisted suicide is illegal, without having a reason for thinking that the laws affect the physician's obligations, then their advice is not ethical advice at all, but rather mere legal advice.[43] In order for the law to play any role at all in their recommendations, they will need to know the moral status of laws. In the case that assisted suicide is illegal in some jurisdiction, an ethicist cannot give all-things-considered advice unless the ethicists happens to recommend against assisting in the suicide for reasons completely unrelated to its legal status. In any other case, the ethicist will need to consider the moral significance of the law.

Others take a more modest view of the role of the clinical ethicist, portraying the clinical ethicist as someone whose work is to give nondirective services, such as analysis of ethical problems, explanation of relevant ethical theory, and discussion of ethical options.[44] If such an adviser is to provide help adequate for determining what is ethical he or she must be able, at a minimum, to clarify why the existence of laws regulating some aspect of clinical practice might or might not be thought to make a difference to the ethics of some case.

In cases where options for clinical practice are constrained by law or policy—which is to say, in nearly all cases—then, considering the moral significance of laws and policies is a crucial task for clinical ethics, and it implicitly undergirds much clinical ethics advice. And, to understand the moral significance of laws, we must at a minimum understand what justifies laws and policies. So, whether bioethicists act as policy advisers or clinical ethicists, it seems that one crucial task for bioethics will be giving an account of what justifies law and policy.

HOW TO JUSTIFY LAW AND POLICY

Ideal Normative Arguments Relating to Law and Policy

Bioethics, then, has at least two major political tasks: making normative recommendations for laws and policies, and making ethics recommendations in a clinical context that is heavily regulated by law and policy. Furthermore, bioethics—particularly philosophical bioethics—is in the business of giving arguments for the recommendations that it makes. But what sort of argument could justify a normative recommendation for law or policy? And what sort of argument could justify an ethical recommendation to either obey or disobey existing legal regulations? In what follows, I will show why either question requires some input from what is best described as normative political philosophy.

First, consider what sort of argument could justify a law or policy. As I mentioned earlier, the arguments given in support of laws or policies often—perhaps usually—focus on the nature or qualities of the actions that those laws or policies target. For example, debate around topics like abortion and euthanasia almost always begin with a discussion of the morality of abortion and euthanasia. However, when we think about justifying a *law*, it is not the actions that the law targets that stand in need of justification: it is the actions associated with passing and enforcing the law that stand in need of justification. Assessing law or policy often proceeds by evaluating the *content* of the law or policy, which naturally lends itself to thinking about the actions that are targeted by the law—whether they are good or bad, etc. To avoid making this mistake it will help us to understand laws and policies not as documents but instead as the actions of political actors such as governments (or more distally, the citizens they represent in a democracy), who pass and enforce those laws.

Suppose then we want to know whether a law treating some action X (such as abortion or euthanasia) in some manner M (for example, prohibited, mandated, incentivized, etc) is justified. In that case, what we want to know is whether the government (or voters, exercising political agency through the government) should or can treat X in M. So, the thing to be justified will not be the law or policy per se, but instead the government's action of treating X in manner M.

What sort of argument could justify the government treating X in manner M? We might start with a moral judgment that X is of moral quality

Q (immoral, virtuous, unjust, contrary to duty, morally required, etc.), but we will need an additional premise if we want to conclude from this that X should/can be treated in manner M. Consider:

Case 1: Moral judgment grounds a law

Major premise$_1$: Actions/states of affairs of moral quality Q should/can be treated in manner M by governments

Minor premise$_1$: X is of moral quality Q

Conclusion$_1$: X should/can be treated in manner M by the government

The first premise is strictly necessary for reaching the conclusion. It is not clear how it is possible to reach a conclusion of the type presented here without relying, at least implicitly, on some general premise similar to the major premise in the syllogism above about what governments can or should do.

In much the same way we can also consider what sort of argument could theoretically justify an ethical recommendation to either obey or disobey a law. Here, the thing to be explained is the moral judgment that some action X has some moral quality, Q, by virtue of (or perhaps, despite) the fact that it has been treated in some manner, M, by law. So:

Case 2: Legality grounds a moral judgment

Major premise$_2$: The government's treatment of an action or state of affairs in manner M gives (or fails to give) that action/state of affairs moral quality Q

Minor premise$_2$: X is treated in manner M by the government

Conclusion$_2$: Therefore, X is (or is not) of moral quality Q

This syllogism is essentially the inverse of Case 1. Instead of beginning with a judgment about the moral quality of Q, it attempts to reach a judgment about the moral quality of Q in light of existing legislation or policy regulating Q. So, we might imagine again a physician considering a request for physician-assisted suicide (PAS). In most jurisdictions, PAS is still illegal. The conclusion that PAS is *consequently* morally impermissible can only be made if we elicit some additional premise about the government's authority, some premise that by making it illegal, it is also immoral. This premise appears as major premise$_2$ in the syllogism above, in a way similar to Case 1.

Of course, it may not always be desirable to assess the morality of an action in an all-things-considered sense. It is perfectly possible to ask whether PAS is morally permissible in abstraction from how existing laws or policies treat it. But, as I argued earlier, it seems necessary for clinical ethicists to consider the moral relevance of law and policy because PAS is illegal in most jurisdictions. Assuming that clinical ethicists give practical ethical advice for actual decisions, they must presumably take into account whether existing legislation alters the ethics of PAS in some way.

The Missing Premise and the Job of Political Philosophy

The major premise, in both syllogisms above, is a general and normative premise relating to governmental action—in Case 1, what justifies governmental actions, and in Case 2, the moral implications of governmental actions.

Broadly speaking, political philosophy is the discipline most directly concerned with studying normative claims related to the government. John Simmons captures this idea when he defines political philosophy as the "evaluative study of political societies," where a political society is a "society with a functioning government."[45] However, this may be too broad since it is possible to evaluate political societies in ways unrelated to their political aspects (for example, we might evaluate whether those living in Mexico eat too many or too few pancakes). So, it seems like a definition is better if it focuses on governments[46] specifically. For this reason, I prefer Narveson's definition: political philosophy is simply a "normative inquiry" asking "what makes government just or legitimate or good."[47] This definition may not seem to capture the question of Case 2, namely, the question about the moral implications of laws and policies—for example, whether there is a duty to obey the government. However, an account of what makes government just or legitimate or good will generally go a long way toward settling whether there is also a duty to obey, since whatever makes government just, legitimate, or good (if anything does) will usually explain (at least in part) why and to what extent people are bound to obey it. It also does not seem possible to answer the question about duties to obey without first considering what makes government just or legitimate or good. Political philosophy, then, as a normative inquiry into what makes government just or legitimate or good, is where we should look for accounts of the second premise listed in each of Cases 1 and 2 above.

Major premise$_1$: Actions/states of affairs of moral quality Q should/can be treated in manner M by governments

Major premise$_2$: The government's treatment of an action/state of affairs in manner M gives (or fails to give) that action/state of affairs moral quality Q

CONCLUSION

Bioethics is fundamentally concerned with normatively justifying laws and policies, whether we consider the field as the dispenser of policy advice, the producer of scholarship touching on law and policy, or the source of clinical ethics advice in a legally regulated context. Normative justification of laws and policies depends, however, on premises about what governments should do; and political philosophy deals with such premises by giving general accounts about what makes government just or legitimate or good. Does bioethics consequently utilize normative political philosophy or directly address general and normative questions about governments? It is to that question we now turn.

NOTES

1. I am indebted to Nathaniel Brown, MD, PhD for advice relating to the plausibility and medical aspects of this imaginary case.
2. By "law," I will mean roughly legislation, understood in light of subsequent authoritative judicial interpretation, where it exists. By "policy," I mean something broader—the government's way of approaching various tasks related to exercising its official functions. Policy can thus include things like an intentional decision to selectively enforce certain kinds of laws, such as laws against possession of even small amounts of marijuana, or laws prohibiting jaywalking. It can also include various rules created as administrative law, which reflect the distinctive emphases of different administrations and can exert significant influence over the real function of government. For more discussion, see Theodore J Lowi, "Law Vs. Public Policy: A Critical Exploration," *Cornell Journal of Law and Public Policy* 12, no. 3 (2003). By using the terms "law and policy" together, I intend to designate all the government's activities involved in the exercise of political power.
3. The idea that patients, rather than physicians or others, have a right to make their own decisions can be traced at least to *Schloendorff v. Society of New York Hospital*, 105 N. E. 92 (N.Y. 1914).
4. President's Commission for the Study of Ethical Problems in Medicine and Biomedical and Behavioral Research, *Deciding to Forego Life-Sustaining Treatment: A Report on the Ethical, Medical, and Legal Issues in Treatment Decisions* (Washington, DC: U.S. G.P.O., 1983).
5. While the majority of commissioners were not bioethicists, the work on the distinctions between acts of omission and commission and the moral differences between withholding and withdrawing care were largely the result of commissioned essays by moral philosophers Dan Brock and Allen Buchanan. Albert R. Jonsen, *The Birth of Bioethics* (New York: Oxford University Press, 1998), 112.
6. President's Commission, *Deciding to Forego*, 89.

7. W. J. Chon et al., "When the Living and the Deceased Cannot Agree on Organ Donation: A Survey of Us Organ Procurement Organizations (OPOS)," *American Journal of Transplantation* 14, no. 1 (2014). Alexandra K Glazier, "Organ Donation and the Principles of Gift Law," *Clinical Journal of the American Society of Nephrology* 13, no. 8 (2018).

8. President's Commission for the Study of Ethical Problems in Medicine and Biomedical and Behavioral Research, *Defining Death: A Report on the Medical, Legal and Ethical Issues in the Determination of Death* (Washington, D.C.: U.S. G.P.O., 1981).

9. National Conference of Commissioners on Uniform State Laws, "Uniform Determination of Death Act," (1980).

10. Kidney sales are illegal in most jurisdictions. However, after Iran legalized the sale of kidneys it eliminated its waiting list in eleven years. Ahad J. Ghods and Shekoufeh Savaj, "Iranian Model of Paid and Regulated Living-Unrelated Kidney Donation," *Clinical Journal of the American Society of Nephrology* 1, no. 6 (2006).

11. "Ethical Principles in the Allocation of Human Organs," accessed 9/21/21, https://optn.transplant.hrsa.gov/resources/ethics/ethical-principles-in-the-allocation-of-human-organs.

12. Van Rensselaer Potter, "Bioethics, the Science of Survival," *Perspectives in Biology and Medicine* 14, no. 1 (1970).

13. For the story of the "bilocated birth" of the term, see W. T. Reich, "The Word "Bioethics": Its Birth and the Legacies of Those Who Shaped It," *Kennedy Institute of Ethics Journal* 4, no. 4 (1994); Warren Thomas Reich, "The Word "Bioethics": The Struggle over Its Earliest Meanings," *Kennedy Institute of Ethics Journal* 5, no. 1 (1995).

14. It was originally called The Institute of Society, Ethics and the Life Sciences.

15. Albert R Jonsen, "A History of Bioethics as Discipline and Discourse," in *Bioethics: An Introduction to the History, Methods, and Practice*, ed. N. A. S. Jecker, A. R. Jonsen, and R. A. Pearlman (Jones and Bartlett Publishers, 2007).

16. Jonsen, *The Birth of Bioethics*, 325.

17. Daniel Callahan, *Abortion: Law, Choice and Morality*, (New York: Macmillan, 1970).

18. Jonsen, *The Birth of Bioethics*, 22.

19. Jonsen, *The Birth of Bioethics*, 21.

20. John Hyde Evans, *Playing God? Human Genetic Engineering and the Rationalization of Public Bioethical Debate* (Chicago: University of Chicago Press, 2002), 89.

21. Discussed in Jonsen, *The Birth of Bioethics*, 23. Charles E. Curran, *Politics, Medicine, and Christian Ethics: A Dialogue with Paul Ramsey* (Philadelphia: Fortress Press, 1973); G. Outka, "Social Justice and Equal Access to Health Care," *The Journal of Religious Ethics* 2, no. 1 (1974).

22. Jonsen, *The Birth of Bioethics*, 98.

23. The National Commission for the Protection of Human Subjects of Biomedical and Behavioral Research. *Belmont Report*. Washington, DC: U.S. Department of Health and Human Services. 1979.

24. Department of Health, Education and Welfare, "45 CFR 46. Protection of Human Subjects," *Federal Register* 39, no. 105 (1974).

25. Bradford H. Gray, "Bioethics Commissions: What Can We Learn from Past Successes and Failures?," in *Society's Choices: Social and Ethical Decision Making in Biomedicine*, ed. Ruth Ellen. Bulger, Elizabeth Meyer. Bobby, and Harvey V. Fineberg (Washington, D.C.: National Academy Press, 1995).

26. Baruch A. Brody, "Limiting Life-Prolonging Medical Treatment: A Comparative Analysis of the President's Commission and the New York State Task Force," in *Society's Choices Social and Ethical Decision Making in Biomedicine*, ed. Ruth Ellen. Bulger et al. (Washington, D.C.: National Academy Press, 1995).

27. For a list, see https://bioethicsarchive.georgetown.edu/pcsbi/former-commissions.html.

28. Obama appointed Amy Gutmann as the chair of his advisory panel on Nov. 25, 2009.

29. For recent examples, see: Eli Y. Adashi and I. Glenn Cohen, "An Overdue Executive Order: Reinstating the National Bioethics Commission," *The American Journal of Medicine* (2021); The Association of Bioethics Program Directors, "Letter to President Biden," (5/24/21 2021). https://www.bioethicsdirectors.net/wp-content/uploads/2021/06/ABPD-letter-Presidential-Bioethics-Commission.pdf.

30. Evans, *Playing God? Human Genetic Engineering and the Rationalization of Public Bioethical Debate*.

31. Evans, *Playing God? Human Genetic Engineering and the Rationalization of Public Bioethical Debate*, 136.

32. Evans, *Playing God? Human Genetic Engineering and the Rationalization of Public Bioethical Debate*, 135.

33. Evans, *Playing God? Human Genetic Engineering and the Rationalization of Public Bioethical Debate*, 144–45.

34. Evans, *Playing God? Human Genetic Engineering and the Rationalization of Public Bioethical Debate*, 151.

35. Bonnie Steinbock, John Arras, and Alex John London, *Ethical Issues in Modern Medicine*, 6th ed. (Boston: McGraw-Hill, 2003).

36. Leonard H. Glantz et al., "Research in Developing Countries: Taking Benefit Seriously," in *Ethical Issues in Modern Medicine*, ed. Bonnie Steinbock, John Arras, and Alex John London (Boston: McGraw-Hill, 2003), 781.

37. Ezekiel J. Emanuel and Linda L. Emanuel, "Four Models of the Physician-Patient Relationship," in *Ethical Issues in Modern Medicine*, ed. Bonnie Steinbock, John Arras, and Alex John London (Boston: McGraw-Hill, 2003), 67.

38. For example, Tom L. Beauchamp, *Contemporary Issues in Bioethics*, 7th ed, (United States: Thomson/Wadsworth, 2008); David DeGrazia, Thomas A. Mappes, and Jeffrey Brand-Ballard, *Biomedical Ethics* (New York: McGraw-Hill Higher Education, 2011).

39. For example, consider an early and widely anthologized article by James Rachels ("Active and Passive Euthanasia," *The New England Journal of Medicine* 292, no. 2 (1975).). Rachels's ostensible subject was a recent statement by the AMA condemning euthanasia. Rachels considers whether there is a morally important

distinction between killing and letting die and argues that there is not. Even so, at the end of the article Rachels considers whether his argument matters; after all, euthanasia and assisted suicide were at that time illegal in all U.S. jurisdictions. Says Rachels, "doctors . . . should . . . be concerned with the fact that the law is forcing upon them a moral doctrine that may well be indefensible and has a considerable effect on their practices." Rachels clearly thinks the legal implications of his argument are, at least in their major effect, obvious; and he seems to hope his argument convinces physicians that laws criminalizing such killings are wrongheaded, despite never specifically saying this.

40. Ruth R. Faden and Tom L. Beauchamp, *A History and Theory of Informed Consent* (New York: Oxford University Press, 1986), 284.

41. Ezekiel J. Emanuel, *The Ends of Human Life: Medical Ethics in a Liberal Polity* (Cambridge, MA: Harvard University Press, 1991), 23.

42. For examples, see Francoise Baylis, "Persons with Moral Expertise and Moral Experts: Wherein Lies the Difference?," in *Clinical Ethics: Theory and Practice*, ed. C. Barry Hoffmaster, Benjamin Freedman, and Gwen Fraser (Clifton, N.J.: Humana Press, 1989); Francoise C Baylis, "The Health Care Ethics Consultant," *Human Studies* 22, no. 1 (1999); Susan B. Sherwin and F. Baylis, "The Feminist Health Care Ethics Consultant as Architect and Advocate," *Public Affairs Quarterly* 17, no. 2 (2003); Abram Brummett and Christopher J Ostertag, "Two Troubling Trends in the Conversation over Whether Clinical Ethics Consultants Have Ethics Expertise," *HEC Forum* 30, no. 2 (2017).

43. Because clinical ethics has been so heavily affected by existing laws and regulations, clinical ethicists often play an informal role in advising practitioners about the legal acceptability of various options in relevant cases. For this reason, one commentator argues that the value of clinical ethics is in part that it provides "inexpensive, on-the-spot, legal advice." H. Tristram Engelhardt, "Why Clinical Bioethics So Rarely Gives Morally Normative Guidance," in *Bioethics Critically Reconsidered: Having Second Thoughts*, ed. H. Tristram Engelhardt (Dordrecht: Springer, 2012).

44. David J. Casarett, Frona Daskal, and John Lantos, "The Authority of the Clinical Ethicist," *Hastings Center Report* 28, no. 6 (1998); Engelhardt, "Why Clinical Bioethics So Rarely Gives Morally Normative Guidance."; Ana S Iltis and Mark Sheehan, "Expertise, Ethics Expertise, and Clinical Ethics Consultation: Achieving Terminological Clarity," *The Journal of Medicine and Philosophy* 41, no. 4 (2016); Lisa M. Rasmussen, "Clinical Ethics Consultants Are Not "Ethics" Experts—but They Do Have Expertise," *The Journal of Medicine and Philosophy* 41, no. 4 (2016).

45. A. John Simmons, *Political Philosophy* (New York: Oxford University Press, 2008), 1, 8.

46. The terms "government" and "state" are sometimes used interchangeably. When they are distinguished, the "state" is often considered as the full set of legal and political institutions in a political community, while the "government" is the persons currently controlling those institutions. Consequently, it is the government that makes laws and can be subject to norms and principles of political philosophy, in a way that a set of institutions usually can not. However, Kant uses the term "government" to

refer to the executive branch in contrast to legislative and judicial branches (6:316), but the term "state" when referring to the entire political community (6:313). I generally prefer to use the terms in their contemporary sense, although sometimes I will use the term "state" when explaining Kant's theory, even though I would ordinarily use "government." Sharply distinguishing between the terms will not typically be important for the purposes of the present work.

47. Jan Narveson, *You and the State: A Fairly Brief Introduction to Political Philosophy* (Lanham: Rowman & Littlefield Publishers, 2008), 11.

Chapter 2

Bioethics and Its Political Philosophy Problem

INTRODUCTION

Although the field of bioethics is inherently political, on the whole bioethics has spent little time engaging with political philosophy,[1] that is, with accounts about what makes government good, just, or legitimate. In this chapter, I will document this neglect. I will also give an account about how it originated, and how it has subsequently caused significant problems in the way the field approaches issues of law and policy.

The purpose of this chapter is to investigate the tools that bioethics typically uses to address political issues, and to make a very general claim about the insufficiency of the tools usually employed in the field. But it is important to qualify these aims by remembering that bioethicists are a diverse bunch who have major disagreements about the methods and theories and aims that should characterize the field. Some individual authors make extensive use of political philosophy in their work, while others have theoretical commitments that essentially preclude treating political philosophy as importantly different from moral philosophy.

Even so, we can make general characterizations of the field by looking at mainstream and widely cited works. From these, we can discern some of the field's shared assumptions about how to approach law and policy, as well as background assumptions about the proper place of theory. My aim here is to illustrate and question some of these widely shared assumptions. In short, I think that bioethics is committed to a modest role for moral theory, and that this commitment, modest as it is, cannot be squared with the way the field typically justifies laws and policies.

I intend this chapter to provide the general context for the more specific problems I will show with the Kantian bioethics literature in later chapters. The problems with the Kantian bioethics literature must be understood in the context of problems with the whole field. Conversely, the problems of the whole field can be illustrated concisely by showing the incoherence of Kantian treatments of law and policy. Together, these descriptions show why bioethics needs to begin incorporating political philosophy in its prescriptions for law and policy.

THE EMERGENCE OF BIOETHICS THEORY

The Problem of Pluralism in Group Decision Making

Understanding the way that bioethicists have thought and do think about the role of theory requires a brief excursion into the history of the field.

Over the course of the 20th century, biomedical technology developed at a rate that would have been previously inconceivable. In chapter 1, I mentioned some of the innovations that prompted new ethical problems: mechanical ventilators, dialysis machines, organ transplant procedures, and technologies that allowed direct observation and even manipulation of the human genome. At the same time, social developments also accelerated changes in the practice of medicine and biomedical research. The heightened capabilities of new medical technologies made health care an increasingly important good, but new technologies were often expensive and scarce, which prompted questions about how best to arrange access to health care. Standardization and regulation of the medical profession, as well as the emergence of new forms of physician labor organization (increasingly in group practices), raised new questions about the relationship between physicians and their employers, about their duties to patients (who might have access to a limited number of physicians through insurance plans or government allocation schemes), and about the regulations that governed the profession. Health research became an increasingly important area of social and governmental investment. These changes prompted many people to ask novel moral questions, or (depending on how one looks at it) old moral questions about new developments in new circumstances.

Despite the changes that made ethical reflection seem increasingly important, a significant problem attended developing answers to the questions posed by these changes. This was the problem of moral pluralism. Moral pluralism was particularly associated with religious diversity, and competing theological traditions had, by this point, been the major contributors to the incipient literature addressing bioethical issues.[2] It was also a feature of the developed literature on philosophical ethics. Although philosophers had not engaged much in practical ethics at this point,[3] normative ethics (that is, the study of ethical theories) was, by the time of the 1970s, largely divided between proponents of consequentialist theory (such as utilitarians) and deontological theory (such as Kantians).

Background pluralism by itself is not an obstacle to ethical decision making. But because medicine and health research were increasingly practiced in a context of social coordination, "ethical" decisions increasingly had to be made in group contexts—for example, by institutional research ethics committees, hospital committees, or government commissions. Moreover, the institutional context of these decisions also meant that their decisions would often affect multiple parties in various ways. A hospital ethics committee decision might set a precedent and so bind all the physicians working at that hospital, as well as patients with limited access to other hospitals, for example. This changing social context of ethical decision making posed a problem because for any decision, one could expect a plurality of views about morality—both within the groups making decisions, and also among those who were affected by them.

Principles as the Solution

It was in this context that Congress called the first government commission on bioethics in 1973—the Belmont Commission, discussed briefly in the last chapter—asking them to "identify basic ethical principles" for the use of human subjects in research. Stephen Toulmin, a staff member on the Commission, recounts that one commentator mentioned cynically that they would see "matters of eternal principle decided by a six to five vote."[4] But according to Toulmin, the Commission actually had a relatively easy time coming to conclusions on many practical matters, despite the existence of background pluralism. The Commission found that they had a great deal of agreement on specific cases, but they got into intractable debates when they tried to go further than this and explain why resolutions to various cases were ethically correct. The Commission decided it could recommend a set of principles, "among those generally accepted within our cultural tradition,"[5] that could guide ethical decision making and satisfy the mandate. The principles espoused in the Report (respect for persons, beneficence, and justice) were consequently mid-level, in the sense that they were general enough to guide decision making on a range of moral issues, but not so general as to give answers to foundational questions about what ultimately makes an action right or wrong, good or bad.

At the same time, two scholars and friends at Georgetown University—Tom Beauchamp and James Childress—had begun work on a groundbreaking book, *Principles of Biomedical Ethics*. They recount that at the time, they understood philosophical ethics as characterized by a deadlock between consequentialist and deontological ethics. Beauchamp was inclined more toward rule consequentialist ethics and Childress toward deontological ethics. But, in their words,

> We quickly realized that our different approaches could generate and sustain a common set of ethical principles for bioethical discourse and practice. This insight is probably the true beginning of *Principles of Biomedical Ethics*. We appreciated the need for an approach that recognized the value of ethical theory for practical judgments but that did not fetishize a single type of theory or promote a single principle over all others.[6]

The "common set of principles" they developed contained four mid-level principles: respect for autonomy, beneficence, non-maleficence, and justice.

While they were writing, both were called to participate in the Belmont Commission. Beauchamp, although not a commissioner, was eventually asked to author the *Belmont Report* and recounts how he moved back and forth between working on the government report and the manuscript for *Principles*. However, despite the similarity between the two sets of principles developed in the report and the manuscript, and the fact that Beauchamp and Childress both worked on both projects, according to Beauchamp the two sets of principles were conceived independently.[7] Assuming this is true, it attests to the common perception among scholars at that time about both the problem that needed solving (a problem of pluralism for decision making in group contexts) and the best way in which to do it (a set of common mid-level principles).

The importance of both the *Belmont Report* and *Principles* for the nascent field could hardly be overestimated. As we noted in the last chapter, the *Belmont Report* served as the foundation for the Common Rule, which continues to regulate the functions of IRBs and consequently all research at institutions accepting U.S. federal funding. And *Principles* did, as Jonsen explains, "set the agenda" for the next decade.[8] It seems likely that the influence of the two documents was reciprocal: federal regulations made learning the "principles" approach mandatory for all those serving on IRBs and, to a lesser extent, for all scientists proposing research governed by these bodies. And *Principles* gave a theoretical and scholarly backing to the Belmont principles that made them a respectable object of study for the classroom and for invocation in the bioethics literature.

BIOETHICS THEORY ON LAW AND POLICY

The problem confronting early bioethicists, as I have portrayed it, appeared to them as a problem requiring a theory or method that could be applied in a variety of group settings where health care ethics decisions are made, without invoking the problems characteristic of moral pluralism.

Beauchamp and Childress were among the first to try to solve this problem, but the basic features of their solution, although contributing to its success, also had significant effects on the way in which they subsequently treated issues of law and policy. I will argue that the problem as they perceived it required a set of principles that could identify primary moral duties while remaining abstract enough that these could be applied to any group making decisions, including groups as diverse as physicians and governments. However, their approach creates special problems when applied to governments, because it encourages the idea that laws should enforce morality; misconstrues political philosophy as relevant primarily for settling the content of our moral duties; and obscures significant moral distinctions between very different kinds of moral agents, such as physicians and governments.

In this section, I will give an overview of the theory proposed by Beauchamp and Childress as solution to the problem of the 1960s and 1970s, and I will describe how their solution lends itself to a problematic approach to issues of law and policy. This section will be somewhat detailed, both because of the importance of Beauchamp and Childress's theory, and also because we will use the problems with their treatment as a template for showing similar problems in other accounts.

Principlism

Principles of Biomedical Ethics

As already noted, in *Principles* Beauchamp and Childress present four ethical principles (respect for autonomy, beneficence, non-maleficence, and justice). These four principles require persons to respect and support autonomous decisions; to avoid causing harm; to provide benefits and relieve harm; and to fairly distribute benefits and costs, respectively.[9] These principles, according to them, compose the part of the "common morality" most relevant to problems in biomedical ethics. The common morality to which they refer is the "set of universal norms shared by all persons committed to morality."[10] These norms have developed through the course of history and are widely shared across cultures—so they have an empirical basis—while also being normatively binding.[11] The four principles are prima facie binding, in the sense that they ordinarily bind us in the absence of countervailing moral principles. Because the four principles are somewhat general, operating at a mid-level principles, they can only be applied in concrete situations through a process of specification. Specification adds content to general norms to make them applicable to particular cases. For example, Beauchamp and Childress offer that the respect for autonomy principle might be specified with respect to advance directives to produce a rule such as, "respect the autonomy of competent patients by following their advance directives when they become incompetent."[12] This is only one way of specifying the general norm, and even this specific rule may need further specification in some circumstances. Although it is the general principles that compose the common morality, specifications of these principles in various rules may also be universally accepted and so become part of the common morality.[13] On the other hand, sometimes specifications are only accepted by a subset of persons, in which case they constitute particular moralities.

Appropriate specification of norms does not necessarily guarantee that it will be clear what to do when faced with an ethical decision. Sometimes proper specification of norms makes clear that a decision requires a choice between conflicting prima facie norms themselves. This is called a moral dilemma. Moral dilemmas are typically resolved through a process of "balancing," in which the person solving the moral dilemma must find reasons for letting one of the prima facie norms prevail, subsequently infringing on one or more others.

How did this theory solve the problem of pluralism in medical decision making? The answer is found in the idea that the four principles are mid-level principles that avoid the polarizing claims of traditional moral theories, and the subsequent addition to their theory of the claim that these principles are also part of a universal common morality.[14] Beauchamp and Childress argue that there is an important difference between principlism and classical theories of normative ethics (such as utilitarianism or Kantianism) that had been the source of ethical pluralism: namely, classical theories purport to explain the foundation or basis of moral obligation, while the principlist theory seeks only to describe mid-level "action-guiding principles" that are widely accepted among morally serious persons.[15] These action-guiding principles are contained in "pre-theoretical" morality, and are the rules and principles that classical moral theories are generally designed to explain and on which they "converge."[16] The common morality thus contains the four principles, but also many more specific rules encountered nearly universally across cultures and times, such as "do not kill," "tell the truth," "nurture the young and dependent," etc.[17] It is in this way, then, that the principlist approach can purport to be a method capable of justifying decisions even in the presence of plural competing philosophical and theological ethical views. The common morality can be the basis for deliberation, justification, and consensus without bogging participants down in divisive questions about the ultimate foundations of ethical truth.

Understanding the Scope of Principlism: Primary Moral Duties

Although the four principles operate at one level of abstraction down from traditional moral theories, they have one important feature in common with them: they are theories of primary, rather than secondary, moral duties and rights.

The distinction I mean to draw between theories of primary moral duties and rights and theories of secondary ones is roughly the distinction between theories about what we owe directly to each other, and theories about how we may (or must) coerce, incentivize, or otherwise influence others who may not do what they are supposed to. This distinction is intended to correspond to the difference between "first order" and "second order" moral questions discussed in chapter 1. Primary moral rights on most views include our basic rights not to be killed, injured, or stolen from; primary moral duties on most views include our duties corresponding to the rights of others, but also usually include duties to act beneficently, fairly, or in ways that avoid unnecessarily harming the interests of others even when they have no right to this. Secondary moral rights might include rights to threaten, coerce, or incentivize others to respect our moral rights, or perhaps a duty to form a government that can protect the rights of others or ensure distributive justice. The right not to be a victim of theft is a primary right; the right to forcefully reclaim what is mine from a thief is a secondary one.

Primary rights and duties are the focus of classical moral theories, and also the focus of the principlist account. Classical moral theories propose answers to questions about the moral obligations of individual persons. For example, Kantian deontology holds that we have certain duties, prescribed by practical reason, that are obligatory. Kant develops a laundry list of these duties in his moral works, especially the *Doctrine of Virtue*: on his account, moral principles categorically proscribe a variety of actions including lying and suicide; positively, they require acting charitably, and developing one's own moral powers, skills, and talents, among other things.

Secondary rights and duties are often the domain of political philosophy. While political theories often assume an underlying account of primary moral duties and rights to some extent, a theory about how we should or may respond when others fail to fulfill their primary moral duties raises special issues. An account of our secondary rights and duties may not follow in a direct or obvious way from the underlying account about primary moral duties. For example, elements of Kantian moral theory have been used as a basis for a variety of competing political philosophies, including

Nozick's libertarianism,[18] Rawls's liberal egalitarianism,[19] Wolff's anarchy,[20] and Kant's own distinctive brand of liberal deontology (a version of which I will develop in chapters five through eight). Other moral theories are similar. Utilitarianism holds that the morality of an action is determined by the extent to which it promotes happiness and minimizes unhappiness. But this view does not directly yield an account of secondary duties or rights. Mill (perhaps the most influential proponent of utilitarianism) thought that utilitarianism suggested that governments should strictly refrain from interfering in actions that do not harm others, even when these harm oneself or appear to be immoral.[21] On the other hand, subsequent utilitarians have often been more sanguine about interfering with self-harming activities if such interference can plausibly maximize happiness. There is no one-to-one relationship between moral and political theories because the question about how we should or may influence the behavior of others—whether to prevent them from violating their moral duties, or to incentivize them to act in desirable ways—is not reducible to the question about how *they* should be acting. As discussed in chapter 1, government intervention in various health-related activities can only be justified by answering basic questions about what governments should do, even if the answers to those questions are in some way conditioned on answers to questions about the moral justifiability of the actions in which they intervene.

Beauchamp and Childress's principlism is firmly in the "primary moral duty" camp. This focus is no doubt in part because many of the questions that they hoped to answer were questions about how physicians, health researchers, or other health care professionals should behave toward patients, subjects, etc. Since physicians and health researchers do not, ordinarily, try to control patients or other persons, a focus on primary moral duties makes most sense for application to these groups.

That their theory is designed to address moral rather than political problems is reinforced by their discussion of theory in *Principles*. In short, they view their theory as a competitor to other basic moral theories that outline primary moral duties, rather than to political theories.[22] So, their discussion of the theories that compete with their own is a discussion of theories of primary moral duties: utilitarian theory, Kantian theory, rights theory, and virtue theory. They discuss each of these theories at length, including a discussion about their strengths and drawbacks. And they apply each of the theories to a case involving a physician trying to decide about whether he has an obligation not to lie to a family on behalf of a father, who could provide an organ transplant to his own dying daughter but has decided that he does not want to. The question is, in other words, about primary moral duties, and the theories are each presented as having relevant answers to this question.

Any of the moral theories they discuss might serve as the embryonic basis for a political theory. But Beauchamp and Childress do not develop any of them in this way. For example, rights theory might sound initially like a political theory. But they consider "rights theory" as a "comprehensive moral theory," not a political theory. And they criticize it as such: it "truncates" morality because it "cannot account for the moral significance of motives, supererogatory actions, virtues, and the like."[23] Further, rights theorists tend to treat "morality's major concern" as protecting "individual rights against governmental . . . intrusion." But, they say, "this vision is too limited for an ethical theory, however it may fare as a political theory." The criticism is telling: their concern is with competing accounts of morality and primary moral duties, not political philosophy. It is the former with which their theory is most usefully compared.[24]

Problems with the Principlist Approach to Law and Policy

Principlism's focus on primary moral duties generates several problems when the theory is applied to issues of law and policy.

Policy as the Enforcement of Moral Duties

First, because Beauchamp and Childress have only a theory of primary duties, law and policy are most naturally evaluated by evaluating the morality of the actions that laws and policies target. This ends up meaning that the purpose of law and morality is effectively understood as enforcing moral duties, albeit with some vague qualifications.

Beauchamp and Childress's basic approach to law and policy is outlined in a short section near the beginning of *Principles*. Here they argue that "moral principles and rules provide a normative structure for policy formation and evaluation."[25] They give various examples of this relationship: for example, they note the importance that moral reflection has had in influencing court decisions about "when artificial devices that sustain life may be withdrawn, whether medically administered nutrition and hydration is a medical treatment that may be discontinued, and whether physicians may be actively involved in hastening a patient's death at the patient's request."[26] The overall import of this discussion, it seems to me, is that the primary metric for judging the moral acceptability of a law is the moral acceptability of the action it regulates.

Do Beauchamp and Childress think that all primary moral duties should be mandated, or violations of these legally prohibited? They qualify their claim about the relationship between law and morality by arguing that it is not inconsistent to hold that something is immoral but should not be prohibited, or that it is moral but need not be mandated.[27] So, evidently not. But they offer no normative principles specific to government that could justify or limit governmental efforts to enforce morality. The reader is consequently left with the impression that governments should generally enforce morality, perhaps with some exceptions.

Political Philosophy and Justice

This is not to say that discussion of principles applying to governments is altogether absent from their work. Beauchamp and Childress do discuss political philosophy in connection with their discussion of the principle of justice. According to Beauchamp and Childress, the principle of justice requires justice in the "distribution of benefits and burdens."[28] They survey six different theories providing various answers to the question about the just distribution of goods (utilitarian, libertarian, egalitarian, communitarian, capability, and well-being theories). These theories, on their treatment, are general theories about how those with resources should distribute them.

By treating political philosophy only in the context of the primary moral duty to distribute benefits and burdens fairly, their treatment suggests—perhaps inadvertently—that political philosophy is mainly relevant for determining the content of our primary moral duties, specifically our duties to distribute goods fairly. This way of treating political philosophy produces two further problems.

First, by treating political philosophy only in the context of the distribution of benefits and burdens, they implicitly suggest—again, perhaps inadvertently—that political philosophy is less relevant to the many issues of law and policy in bioethics (many of which they discuss elsewhere) that are not obviously about the distribution of benefits and burdens. I have already argued that political philosophy is crucial to giving a normative account of law or policy, because normative arguments for law and policy must take a stance on what it is generally legitimate for governments to do. Many law and policy issues in bioethics are not primarily about the distribution of benefits and burdens. For example, governments control licensing among physicians and so control who counts as a medical practitioner (how much training they need, what sorts of competencies they must possess, what disqualifies someone from medical practice), their scope of practice, what counts as malpractice, how physicians may bill, how they may compete with one another, and how they collect, store, and share information about patients. Governments regulate other health professionals in similar ways, from nurses to radiologic technicians. They criminalize the practice of medicine without a license. Governments approve pharmaceuticals and decide who can prescribe them and under what circumstances. Governments criminalize or regulate various kinds of medical procedures, from euthanasia to abortion to the sale of human body parts. They regulate IVF, PGD, and other aspects of medicalized reproduction. They determine who has the authority to make medical decisions, and what constitutes legally valid consent. They engage in original health research. They regulate the health insurance industry by deciding when private companies must accept those with preexisting health conditions, or stipulating that companies must accept high-risk patients, or regulating the kinds of contracts they may write and the kinds of procedures and medications they may or may not choose to exclude from coverage. They can require various kinds of behaviors and procedures to reduce the risk of contracting infectious diseases.

By treating political philosophy only in the constrained context of the distribution of benefits and burdens, Beauchamp and Childress leave us with no specifically political resources for explaining the ethics of government involvement in these other problems. Moreover, because they don't address the general applicability of political philosophy to these issues that obviously involve questions about governmental authority and legitimacy, they further reinforce the idea discussed above that these issues are best resolved by merely enforcing morality.

Second, by eliciting political philosophy only in the context of our primary moral duties, they implicitly suggest (again, perhaps unintentionally) that the duty to fairly distribute benefits and burdens applies in a monolithic way to all kinds of moral agents. On their telling, accounts of justice developed originally as political theories apply variously to researchers selecting subjects for enrollment in research, governments determining whether citizens have a right to health care, and physicians in triage situations deciding who to treat and in what order. Their approach lends itself naturally to this sort of conflation because it focuses on the abstract and primary duty of justice, and so emphasizes the similarity of the duties that are supposedly derived from that principle, rather than the deep moral differences that characterize the agents supposedly bound by it.

But it is implausible to think that the problem of triaging patients is closely related, morally, to the problem of determining whether to create a national right to health care. The fact that they can both be conceived of as distribution problems obscures many of the dissimilarities between them. For example—as I will discuss at more length in chapter 4—one of the characteristic features of governments is that they wield political power, by which I mean they attempt to exercise a monopoly on making, interpreting, and enforcing law within a jurisdiction. In this way, they claim exceptional powers, making them morally different from any other agent within their jurisdiction. When governments determine how to allocate resources, for example, they must first obtain those resources, which they usually do through taxation.

Physicians, in contrast, may also allocate resources, but one of the things they do not characteristically do is raise their funds through taxation. The principle of justice, though, has no particular way of addressing this morally significant difference.[29] If justice tells us about the correct way of distributing resources but has no implications for who distributes them or how those resources are obtained in the first place, then there is no obvious reason why physicians could not set up small private armies to forcibly collect funds for health care from various persons in their geographical area, in a way somewhat analogous to the methods of the state. But this would be ludicrous. What is needed to explain why the principle of justice applies differently to governments than it does to physicians and researchers is a theory of government, a political philosophy. But Beauchamp and Childress do not provide one or discuss political philosophy beyond its limited applicability to distributive issues.[30]

Problems in Action: Principlism on the Legalization of Physician-Assisted Suicide

Several of the problems created by the focus on primary moral duties can be helpfully illustrated by examining Beauchamp and Childress's discussion of the legalization of physician-assisted suicide.

In keeping with their emphasis on primary moral duties, Beauchamp and Childress propose to treat the question about the legalization of assisted suicide as primarily an issue of the *morality* of assisted suicide, a point that they explicitly mention.[31] However, they begin their discussion of assisted suicide with a question about the difference between "acts" and "policies." They argue that there may be reasons to legally prohibit assisted suicide *even if* some cases or acts of assisted suicide are morally permissible. The reasons for this have to do with the potential for "abuse": if the legalization of assisted-suicide will eventually result in loosening of restrictions surrounding assisted suicide, or in changing social mores or attitudes that currently protect vulnerable patients from abuses, then legally prohibiting even morally justified acts of assisted-suicide may be justified.[32]

This discussion of policy clears the ground for the "central question" regarding legalization, which is the question of the morality of assisted suicide.[33] Beauchamp and Childress argue that assisted suicide can be morally justified, for reasons based in the principles of autonomy and beneficence.[34] In their view, the principles of autonomy and non-maleficence justify the withdrawal of life-sustaining treatment from patients suffering from severe illness or pain. According to them, similar considerations also apply to patients who are not dependent on life-sustaining treatment, who can express a competent wish to die (which requires that physicians respect their autonomy) and who are also suffering from severe illness and pain (thus imposing an obligation of beneficence). To allow physicians to end a patient's life[35] in cases where patients rely on life-sustaining treatment but not in cases where they do not would be arbitrary. So, according to Beauchamp and Childress, in cases where the patient's request, the disease, and the "desperateness" of circumstances are all relevantly similar, assisting in death is "morally equivalent" to withdrawing life-sustaining treatment.[36] Laws and policies, they conclude, should attempt to allow such morally justified cases of assisted suicide (they outline a series of "sufficient" conditions defining such cases) while prohibiting morally unjustified cases.[37]

This treatment illustrates two of the problems discussed earlier with their approach to law and policy. First, it is clear, as they admit, that they are centrally concerned with primary duties, specifically, whether there is a moral duty to refrain from assisting in suicide or not. Because the focus is squarely on the primary duty, issues of policy can be treated as effectively derivative issues whose resolution is determined entirely by focusing on the morality of the behavior they would regulate. Preventing a slippery slope that might result in "abuses" may give us practical reasons to prohibit assisted suicide, but this would be the only consideration for law and policy that does not automatically follow from the consideration of the moral status of the action that is the target of law or policy. In other words, the only reason for prohibiting something that is morally legitimate is preventing *other* morally illegitimate actions (i.e., "abuses"). The assumption that assisted suicide should be illegal if it is immoral is apparent but is not defended.

Second, no explicit account of the general moral basis of government regulation of assisted suicide—that is, no political philosophy—is ever given. This illustrates the constrained use of political philosophy in the bioethics literature. Since assisted suicide is not primarily an issue about the distribution of health care, there is no obviously relevant reason to mention the principle of justice or the accounts of political philosophy associated with it. This means we have no general account about when immoral actions should be legally prohibited or why it might be legitimate for governments to criminalize physician involvement in suicide, beyond the bare claims that legalizing assisted suicide might change social views or lead some to commit "abuses."

Other Accounts: Reiterating the Problems of Principlism

Beauchamp and Childress were the first and most influential to attempt a theory of bioethics that could resolve ethical problems in medicine against a backdrop of moral pluralism, but others also sought to solve this problem. Despite offering diverse accounts of morality and method, other major accounts of bioethics theory also share the primary duty focus offered by Beauchamp and Childress, and so share many of the same problems in their approach to law and public policy. Here I will focus on those authors who, like Beauchamp and Childress, are amenable to moral theory in some sense. We will consequently leave aside casuistry and other anti-theory methods of bioethics. The argument I'm advancing is not one for more theory in general, but rather an argument that if one is using theory or principles to solve problems in bioethics, one should use the appropriate kind. I will show that, despite their acceptance of theory and their interest in issues of law and policy, major theoretical approaches to bioethics typically develop only theories of primary moral duties and rarely make constructive use of political philosophy.

Common Morality as a Public System

In a different sort of common morality theory, Gert, Culver, and Clouser propose a theory of morality as a "public system," meaning that the basic content of morality is known by "all those to whom it applies."[38] On their view, morality is composed most basically of moral rules that prohibit actions causing harm to others. Morality does include some other components, including moral ideals about helping others when it is possible, but these do not have the same force as the moral rules.

According to Gert et al., because morality is a public system, it also constitutes a "framework on which all of the disputing parties can agree."[39] The theory thus solves the problem of pluralism by stipulating that, when it comes to the most basic components of morality—the *common* morality—there is no pluralism, because the chief features of this morality are in fact already accepted by everyone.

This solution might seem to solve the problem of pluralism by defining it away. But that is not quite true primarily because Gert et al. do not think that the common morality can solve most—possibly any—of the controversies we associate with moral pluralism. The common morality contains rules that are rarely questioned by anyone. It prohibits, for example, injuring someone without a justifying reason. But it does not solve other problems, such as whether abortion is morally permissible, or what kind of health care system we should have.

Gert et al.'s theory is a theory of primary duties. It purports to explain our common moral duties and presents itself as a competitor to other theories of primary moral duties.[40] It is, as they say, intended primarily as a theory for medical practitioners. They do not offer an account of political philosophy; in contrast to Beauchamp and Childress, they do not even mention theories of distributive justice in their discussion of government-provided health care. On their view, an account of what governments should generally do would "require a whole book."[41] Nevertheless, they still reach normative conclusions about government provision of health care; the legality of abortion; and the legality of physician-assisted suicide and euthanasia, among other things.

The effort they expend on moral theory is impressive; it allows them to reach nuanced positions on metaethics, moral epistemology, normative ethics, and other matters. However, barely a sentence is devoted to the role of the government.[42] If defending a view of governments is too complex a task and the work is directed mostly toward physicians, then arguably they should refrain from taking positions on questions about health care reform or the legality of various medical procedures—which, as I have argued, always require additional premises about what governments should, in general, do.

Feminism

Among the most politically oriented works in bioethics are those written by feminists. These works, while pointing out legitimate shortcomings in mainstream bioethics approaches, also perpetuate some of the same problems in their treatments of law and policy.

Susan Sherwin provides what is perhaps the best-developed feminist theory of bioethics in her book *No Longer Patient*. Sherwin, like those theorists considered earlier, finds traditional theories of ethics (Kantianism, utilitarianism, contractarianism) problematic both because of problems internal to these theories,[43] and also because they are often too abstract to be applied directly to particular cases.[44] Sherwin finds a variety of advantages in methods characteristic of mainstream bioethics (its attention to particular relationships and stories, its understanding of the importance of power differentials such as those between patients and physicians, its reliance on principles rather than abstract theories), but she faults bioethics primarily because its methods do not address, and often obscure, the political context in which various ethical problems occur.

On Sherwin's account, the chief concern of a feminist bioethics is a concern with "the ways in which medicine supports and participates in the complex systems of practices that constitute the oppression of women."[45] Sherwin follows Frye in defining oppression as "an interlocking series of restrictions and barriers that reduce the options available to people on the basis of their membership in a group."[46] Traditional bioethics tends to treat ethical issues by approaching them through isolated cases; if the agents in the case do not violate any rules or ethical principles then bioethicists often decide that the activity is permissible. However, this neglects to consider the overall context in which those practices occur. For example, Sherwin considers how a wide variety of medical practices—everything from surrogacy to cosmetic surgery—while not perhaps objectionable in isolated cases, are ethically problematic when considered against the meaning and role that those practices have in supporting an "interlocking system of harmful practices" that further the oppression and subordination of women.

According to Sherwin, the problem with oppression is that it is unjust.[47] Because oppression has to do with an interlocking web of institutions and practices, and justice is defined primarily in terms of its opposition to oppression, virtually any practice—committed by anyone—can be the target of a justice-based claim, and so be a "political" issue.

The consequence of this is that the feminist theory of health care ethics developed by Sherwin, despite its focus on "politics," oppression, and justice, has at the most only vague normative implications for the government. The problem is similar to the one we noted in connection Beauchamp and Childress's treatment of the principle of justice. Because justice is thought to be a general principle governing all distribution, it has no special implications for governments, and so does not provide a theory of what makes government good, just, or legitimate. Sherwin does, in my view, provide an important lens through which to consider the practices of patients, physicians, researchers, and policymakers; but her view of oppression and the associated concept of justice provides no normative theory about how to make policy and law, beyond asking us to consider the commitments of feminism when making policy. Sherwin seems to admit as much, when she explains that she intends to utilize a kind of "eclectic feminism," that assumes a minimal amount of theory so as to include as many kinds of feminism as possible.[48] But this also limits the extent to which Sherwin's account of feminism can provide normative input into the formation of law and policy.

Deontological Liberalism

Much like the others we have surveyed, H. Tristram Engelhardt seeks to answer the question about whether and to what extent a general secular ethic can resolve moral disputes in a pluralist society. In *The Foundations of Bioethics*, Engelhardt asks whether there exists a canonical secular "content-full morality," that can substantively answer questions about "what is right or wrong, good or bad beyond the very sparse requirements that one may not use others without authorization."[49]

Engelhardt answers this question negatively. In his view, only the thinnest, content-free morality can claim authority over moral strangers (that is, persons who have not or are not willing to acknowledge a source of authority or common method for resolving moral controversies).[50] This content-free morality consists, basically, in a single principle, a "principle of permission." Persons are required to obtain the permission of others before using them, because consent is the only possible basis of a peaceable moral community. This is to say that a principle of permission is something like a condition for the possibility of morals. The concept of morality—and all its associated concepts, like blame- and praise-worthiness—requires that persons be capable of acting freely, that is, capable of choosing to do things because they are morally required.[51] By using force or coercion to bypass the voluntary consent of others, one undermines the conditions that make any kind of moral blame or praise possible. So, permission is a basic necessity for the possibility of morality. For this reason, other moral principles—such as beneficence, non-maleficence, or justice—must be treated as strictly secondary to a principle of permission. According to Engelhardt, allowing "beneficence" to outweigh permission in some situation—such as might occur, for example, in a classic case of paternalism—is effectively to violate the conditions for the possibility of morality on the grounds that one is morally obligated to do so, which is nonsensical. Voluntary commitment to various moral ideals—specific conceptions of beneficence, or of the various distributions sometimes considered requirements of "justice"—are possible, but only in a community of moral friends, i.e., persons committed to similar moral codes or authorities capable of resolving moral controversies, who reside in those communities voluntarily and so effectively give their permission to be governed by the relevant standards or authorities. This is all the moral content that is available to secular moral reason, by which he means moral reason unaided by revelation, intuition, or other unshared premises and assumptions.

Engelhardt, like the others, focuses on primary moral duties, and gives an account of primary moral duties that competes with other moral theories such as Kantianism, utilitarianism, and contractarianism.[52] Moreover, Engelhardt shares some of the problems that typically accompany this focus. For example, he argues that the major obstacle to legal enforcement of various putative moral obligations is the limitations of moral epistemology: if only it were possible to establish a canonical, content-full secular morality, then governments would have the authority to enforce these. But since the existence of these "moral obligations" cannot be established conclusively by reason, governments have no authority to enforce them on those who do not accept them.[53]

Engelhardt's vision of governmental authority to enforce morality differs sharply from the other authors we have considered, in the sense that he thinks governments lack authority to enforce any basically any moral obligations other than the thinnest principle of permission. However, it is important to notice that Engelhardt nevertheless seems to share with these authors the assumption that the existence of a moral obligation not to act in some way is (or would be) sufficient grounds for legally prohibiting it. The difference between Engelhardt's views and those of the others revolve primarily around epistemological issues, regarding whether it is possible to demonstrate the existence of a content-full, secular canonical morality, and not the normative claim that moral duties do, in principle, form the basis for legal requirements. Such an assumption is problematic for reasons we shall consider most carefully in chapter 4, and it obviously relies on an implicit theory of government, which Engelhardt does not further explore.

However, Engelhardt does develop a libertarian account of political philosophy later in a chapter that deals in part with the state.[54] In that chapter Engelhardt surveys a variety of accounts about the basis of political authority, proposes his own account of this based in persons and property, and subsequently discusses the justification of (and limits to) the authority of the state.

It is not clear to me why more bioethicists have not engaged with this discussion about the authority of the state. Engelhardt's libertarian views are not widely shared in bioethics; prominent commentators variously dismiss his theory as "too thin,"[55] "unconvincing,"[56] or going "too far."[57] It is perhaps because his conclusions are widely rejected that commentators have not thought it necessary to propose alternative accounts of the government. In any case, Engelhardt's treatment is an outlier in the bioethics literature because it provides an explicit and normative account of the government.

SURVEYING THE FIELD

The literature developing bioethics theories we have just surveyed is the best place to look when gauging the place generally accorded to political philosophy in bioethics. However, an examination of other genres of bioethics literature, such as introductory texts and works on the relationship between bioethics and the law, further bolsters my claim that political philosophy is missing in important ways from bioethics. Here I will give a brief overview of the approaches to law and policy taken in this literature. We will note that it is very similar to the approach taken in major works of bioethics theory we have already explored, most likely because of the influence of those works.

Introductions and Anthologies

Anthologies and introductions typically contain opening chapters giving some attention to methods, and these chapters virtually always follow the general format pioneered by Beauchamp and Childress in *Principles*. For example, consider the bestselling anthology edited by Lewis Vaughn.[58] Vaughn's introductory chapters are particularly comprehensive, as far as introductory works go, and the discussion of moral theory in chapter 2 is detailed and comprehensive. Although Vaughn does discuss Rawls's theory of justice, it is treated as a contractarian moral theory rather than a theory of government[59] and is considered as a competitor to other theories of morality. Thus, the theories discussed are all moral theories, or theories of primary moral duties as I have called them, and there is no discussion of political theories in the section on theory. Other anthologies and introductory texts follow this same basic pattern in their treatment of theory, with slight variations.[60]

Vaughn, like Beauchamp and Childress, does briefly discuss political philosophy under the principle of justice (he discusses libertarianism and egalitarianism). But here, just as in Beauchamp and Childress, the discussion of political theories is restricted to a single issue—the distribution of health resources—and it is treated as a principle that can apply variously to physicians as well as governments. This suggests, as I have argued, that political philosophy is primarily relevant to distributive issues, and that it applies widely to all those engaged in distributive activities, regardless of whether they represent the government.

Finally, Vaughn does—again, like Beauchamp and Childress—present a very short discussion of the relationship between "morality and the law."[61] Here he points out that saying something is moral is not the same as saying it is legal; just because something is immoral does not necessarily mean it is or should be illegal, and just because something is illegal, does not necessarily mean it is immoral. Like Beauchamp and Childress, however, Vaughn offers no indication about how specifically to determine which things should be illegal, or what the relationship between the two should be. Other anthologies and texts address policy in a similar way.[62]

Bioethics and the Law

It might be expected that materials on bioethics and the law would have a more nuanced approach to explaining the normative basis of laws, but in fact, they typically also follow the methods we have already seen in the bioethics literature.

For example, in a prominent text on law and bioethics, Furrow et al. survey ethical theory. They discuss four theories of ethics (utilitarianism, Kantian theories, religious-based ethics, and natural law), principlism, and three theories they refer to as "contextual theories" (feminist bioethics, critical race theory, and disability theory).[63] All these theories are primarily concerned with what we have described as primary moral duties and rights. There is no discussion of normative theories specifically directed toward government. In the section discussing the relationship between bioethics and law, they give a basically descriptive account of the relationship between ethics and the law. They begin with the commonplace that "law and ethics are not identical," before briefly discussing some of the drawbacks to legislating morality.[64] Then they provide a brief overview about how the law and ethics often share a methodology (case-based reasoning), before pointing out that the law even sometimes incorporates ethical standards (such as the principles in the *Belmont Report* in legislation regulating end-of-life decision making), and that the law sometimes tries to make sure it does not require people to act unethically. But despite much discussion of both the law and theories of morality, they do not discuss general theories of government or what justifies laws.

Similarly, Dolgin and Shepherd follow the discussion of five ethical theories we have already described from Beauchamp and Childress,[65] before going on to describe principlism and critical theory. Their discussion of the relationship between law and bioethics is "historical," showing the variety of ways that bioethics and the law have impacted one another, and they reprint a short essay explaining some of these trends. No normative theories of government or law appear here either.

These sources illustrate the overall approach of this literature, which is best described as normative when it comes to theories of primary ethical duties, but merely descriptive when it discusses the law. Law and bioethics texts may discuss the extent to which law has influenced the field of bioethics;[66] how bioethics literature and thought has been incorporated into law;[67] or whether bioethics can help us to understand the decision making procedures and jurisdictional questions bound up with court decisions.[68] Others attempt to simply give an overview of how existing laws relate to bioethics[69] or compile a series of judicial decisions establishing precedent for traditional bioethics issues.[70] By restricting their discussion of normative theories to theories of primary moral duties, they implicitly suggest that the major problems of justifying law and policy revolve around the ethics of the behaviors that those laws seek to regulate, and they provide no tools for evaluating the ethics of governmental intervention itself.

FINDING POLITICAL PHILOSOPHY IN BIOETHICS

As we have seen, much of bioethics is about law and policy. And, as the discussion so far has indicated, there is no shortage of theory in bioethics. Although some have doubted the importance of theory, theory has been important to many writers in bioethics since the beginning of the field. Even those—especially those—seeking to establish a method that avoids the pitfalls associated with theoretical pluralism have found it important to survey competing ethical theories, and to explain the relationship of their preferred approach to potential competitors. Yet a summary survey of major accounts and overviews found in the literature demonstrates that, while theory is alive and well, accounts of government do not feature in a major way in this literature. In the few cases where political philosophy does play an important role, it is usually invoked to explain the content of our primary moral duties—specifically, our duties to distribute benefits and burdens fairly—rather than to give something like a theory of government that could be applied to issues beyond the distribution of health-related resources. Bioethics, despite its aspirations to give normative guidance for law and policy, has developed almost no resources specific to this task.

I have sought to characterize the dominant strains and approaches to issues of law and policy in the field here. The bioethics literature is growing quickly, and of course there are authors who seek to implement political philosophy or some account of government in their work. By far the largest segment of this work deals with health justice and the allocation of health resources and the social determinants of health. The literature on this topic, which is growing rapidly, sometimes engages with political theory extensively.[71] But the bioethics approach to this topic is often only equivocally political. It is political in the sense that authors assume that accounts of health justice are directly relevant to governments. But its political relevance remains limited in an important way: insofar as it develops only an account of a general and primary duty of justice, it remains unclear what role governments have in distributing health resources. Is the existence of a duty of justice sufficient reason for government intervention? If so, what should be the nature of the government's intervention? Should it force persons to fulfill their duties of justice, or can it fulfill them on their behalf? Is it possible for it to go too far? Showing that justice requires some distribution of resources or pattern of behavior does not by itself answer questions about the laws or policies that governments should implement. Even given an account of justice, political actions cannot be fully normatively justified until we have an account about what makes government good or just or legitimate.

Other topics have also received some attention by those employing specifically political methods, including public health ethics and the literature on bioethicists participating in government commissions.[72] But I will put no further effort into canvassing all these. My claim is not that political philosophy doesn't feature at all in bioethics, but that its importance has been underappreciated by the field. The best evidence for this, in my view, can be seen in the literature applying Kantian philosophy to questions about the legalization of a market in organs, which I will treat in chapter 3.

RIGHTING HEALTH POLICY: RETHINKING POLITICAL PHILOSOPHY IN BIOETHICS

In this chapter I have given a broad and preliminary overview of the place of political philosophy in bioethics. In short, I have argued that political philosophy has barely featured in bioethics. The reasons for this can be traced back to the historical origins of the methods of bioethics and the needs that these methods were designed to address. The approach pioneered in the 1970s is still dominant in theoretical works in bioethics, and has been widely incorporated into introductory materials as well. The approach, whatever its merits for matters of primary moral duties, has severe limitations when applied to law and policy.

However, this preliminary account of bioethics' political philosophy problem is of limited usefulness for two reasons. First, we have only been able to survey major accounts of theory and various kinds of overviews about methods in bioethics. It is possible our evaluation of the bioethics literature would change if we examined the approaches employed by bioethicists working on specific topics concerning law and policy in bioethics. Consequently, in the chapter that follows, we will look in detail at the literature applying Kantian philosophy to questions about legalizing the sale of organs. This will serve as a more in-depth look at dominant patterns in bioethics scholarship.

Second, the question about the importance of political philosophy for reaching conclusions about law and policy is, ultimately, a normative question. There is no "view from nowhere" about what bioethics needs when addressing various problems. I have made a preliminary argument for the importance of political philosophy, but there is no conclusive way to show the importance of theories about what makes government good, just, or legitimate without answering some further questions about morality and the law. Consequently, in the remainder of the book we will address some of these questions in more detail, and I will give an account about why political philosophy is indispensable from at least one perspective, a Kantian one.

NOTES

1. I am not the first to notice the absence of political philosophy in the bioethics literature. See R. Alta Charo, "The Hunting of the Snark: The Moral Status of Embryos, Right-to-Lifers, and Third World Women," *Stanford Law & Policy Review* 6, no. 2 (1995); Richard E. Ashcroft, "Kant, Mill, Durkheim? Trust and Autonomy in Bioethics and Politics," *Studies in History and Philosophy of Biological and Biomedical Sciences* 34, no. 2 (2003); Søren Holm, "Bioethics Down under—Medical Ethics Engages with Political Philosophy," *Journal of Medical Ethics* 31, no. 1 (2005); Jeffrey P. Bishop and Fabrice Jotterand, "Bioethics as Biopolitics," *The Journal of Medicine and Philosophy* 31, no. 3 (2006); Angus Dawson, "Editorial: Political Philosophy and Public Health Ethics," *Public Health Ethics* 2, no. 2 (2009).

2. Albert R. Jonsen, *The Birth of Bioethics* (New York: Oxford University Press, 1998), Ch. 2.

3. Tom Beauchamp and James Childress, "Principles of Biomedical Ethics: Marking Its Fortieth Anniversary," *The American Journal of Bioethics* 19, no. 11 (2019).

4. Stephen Toulmin, "The Tyranny of Principles," *The Hastings Center Report* 11, no. 6 (1981).

5. Jonsen, *The Birth of Bioethics*, 103.

6. Beauchamp and Childress, "Principles of Biomedical Ethics: Marking Its Fortieth Anniversary."

7. Tom L. Beauchamp, "The Origins and Evolution of the Belmont Report," in *Belmont Revisited: Ethical Principles for Research with Human Subjects*, ed. James F. Childress, Eric Mark Meslin, and Harold T. Shapiro (Washington, DC: Georgetown University Press, 2005).

8. Jonsen, *The Birth of Bioethics*, 333.

9. Tom L. Beauchamp and James F. Childress, *Principles of Biomedical Ethics*, 7th ed. (New York: Oxford University Press, 2013), 13.

10. Tom L Beauchamp and James F Childress, *Principles of Biomedical Ethics*, 8th ed. (New York: Oxford University Press, 2019), 3.

11. Beauchamp and Childress, *Principles of Biomedical Ethics*, 8th ed., 4–5.

12. Beauchamp and Childress, *Principles of Biomedical Ethics*, 7th ed., 17.

13. Beauchamp and Childress, *Principles of Biomedical Ethics*, 7th ed., 17.

14. The idea that the principles are part of a "universal common morality" was added in the 3rd edition of their work. See Jennifer Flynn, "Theory and Bioethics," in The Stanford Encyclopedia of Philosophy, ed. Edward N. Zalta (2021). https://plato.stanford.edu/archives/spr2021/entries/theory-bioethics/.

15. Beauchamp and Childress, *Principles of Biomedical Ethics*, 7th ed., 383–84.

16. Beauchamp and Childress, *Principles of Biomedical Ethics*, 7th ed., 383.

17. Tom L. Beauchamp, "The 'Four Principles' Approach to Health Care Ethics," in *Principles of Health Care Ethics*, ed. Richard Edmund Ashcroft et al. (New York: Wiley, 2007).

18. Robert Nozick, *Anarchy, State, and Utopia* (New York: Basic Books, 1974).

19. John Rawls, *A Theory of Justice* (Cambridge, Massachusetts: Belknap Press of Harvard University Press, 1971). Rawls's liberal egalitarianism famously avoids questions about how we should respond when others fail to give us our due. Rawls argues that the basic rules of society should be determined on the assumption that persons know and accept the rules of justice. His theory is in this sense a theory of "ideal" rather than "nonideal" justice. For him, questions about how to deal with non-compliant persons comes at a later stage of political theory (one which he never got around to). Secondary duties and rights are nevertheless still an important question of political philosophy on his account.

20. Robert Paul Wolff, *In Defense of Anarchism* (New York: Harper & Row, 1970).

21. John Stuart Mill, *On Liberty* (New York: Liberal Arts Press, 1956).

22. While Beauchamp and Childress argue that their theory contains only mid-level principles and so is not directly in competition with the moral theories that characteristically compose moral pluralism, they do suggest that other moral theories are limited in their application to public moral problems because they all go beyond the

common morality by committing to methods and sometimes particular moral claims that are not widely accepted. Insofar as Beauchamp and Childress suggest their approach as a replacement to other moral theories, then, their theory is in competition with these—even if only in this qualified sense.

23. Beauchamp and Childress, *Principles of Biomedical Ethics*, 8th ed., 408.

24. Beauchamp and Childress do discuss the possibility that the various ethical theories might be most helpful when applied to a certain range of moral problems. For example, they mention that utilitarianism could perhaps serve as the basis for public policy, because it suggests that we maximize good outcomes for all parties; and that rights theory can serve to protect persons against "unjust or unwarranted communal intrusion, control, or neglect." Although Beauchamp and Childress mention some potential political implications of these theories, they develop them only as theories of morality.

25. Beauchamp and Childress, *Principles of Biomedical Ethics*, 8th ed., 9–10.

26. Beauchamp and Childress, *Principles of Biomedical Ethics*, 8th ed., 9–10.

27. Beauchamp and Childress, *Principles of Biomedical Ethics*, 8th ed., 10.

28. Beauchamp and Childress, *Principles of Biomedical Ethics*, 8th ed., 268.

29. The principlist account arguably creates similar problems when applying the other three principles as well. For example, the principle of beneficence is often deployed to assess the ethics of pediatric decision making. But assessing decisions made by parents, physicians, and the state all from the perspective of the principle of beneficence (expressed in the "best interests standard") arguably obscures some of the important moral differences between these parties in the ways that they relate to children. See D. Robert MacDougall, "Intervention Principles in Pediatric Health Care: The Difference between Physicians and the State," *Theoretical Medicine and Bioethics* 40, no. 4 (2019).

30. "Specification" could theoretically provide an answer to this problem. By specification, Beauchamp and Childress understand a process of reducing the indeterminacy of general norms, such as "justice," to produce more specific rules or principles that give guidance in specific contexts. Specification adds content, and so could theoretically give more determinate rules individualized for governments, researchers, and physicians, developed around their salient moral differences. However, Beauchamp and Childress suggest no rules or principles for application specifically to governments. Doing so would in fact be difficult on their framework, since such a specification would have implications well beyond questions about the distribution of burdens and benefits; consequently, they would have to treat such general principles about governments under each of the principles, presumably. In any case, the point I wish to make is not that principlism *could not* be altered to give a more plausible treatment of the role of government in contrast to other parties. Instead, the point is that by focusing on primary moral duties, it seems natural to omit such a discussion, and to treat the ethics of law and policy as mere extensions of our primary moral duties.

31. Beauchamp and Childress, *Principles of Biomedical Ethics*, 8th ed., 185.

32. Beauchamp and Childress, *Principles of Biomedical Ethics*, 8th ed., 188.

33. Beauchamp and Childress, *Principles of Biomedical Ethics*, 8th ed., 188.

34. See Beauchamp and Childress, *Principles of Biomedical Ethics*, 8th ed., 188.

35. Many persons think that withdrawing care does not kill or end a patient's life, but merely lets the underlying disease take its course. But Beauchamp and Childress argue that this distinction is mistaken, and that the relevant difference between unjustified and justified killings is whether the physician has an obligation not to kill. As they point out, a person who is not a physician who withdraws life-sustaining treatment wrongly would certainly be said to "kill" the patient. Beauchamp and Childress, *Principles of Biomedical Ethics*, 8th ed., 183–84.

36. Beauchamp and Childress, *Principles of Biomedical Ethics*, 8th ed., 192.

37. Beauchamp and Childress, *Principles of Biomedical Ethics*, 8th ed., 192.

38. Bernard Gert, Charles M. Culver, and K. Danner Clouser, *Bioethics: A Systematic Approach*, 2nd ed. (New York: Oxford University Press, 2006), 11.

39. Gert, Culver, and Clouser, *Bioethics: A Systematic Approach*, 2nd ed., 21.

40. See the discussion in chapter 2, on moral disagreement. Gert, Culver, and Clouser, *Bioethics: A Systematic Approach*, 2nd ed.

41. Gert, Culver, and Clouser, *Bioethics: A Systematic Approach*, 2nd ed., 63.

42. The sentence is: "One of the primary responsibilities, if not *the* primary responsibility of government is to lessen the amount of harm suffered by its citizens." Gert, Culver, and Clouser, *Bioethics: A Systematic Approach*, 2nd ed., 63. Since they regard "preventing harm" as an optional moral ideal (p. 43), rather than a nonoptional moral rule, this suggests that they think the government should fulfill our moral ideals for us; but this seems problematic, particularly when doing so requires the government to violate moral rules which are not optional, such as the rule against restricting freedom. Readers should note there is also a short discussion defending the "importance of having public policies." (p. 45).

43. Susan Sherwin, *No Longer Patient: Feminist Ethics and Health Care* (Philadelphia: Temple University Press, 1992), 37–42.

44. Sherwin, *No Longer Patient: Feminist Ethics and Health Care*, 42, 81.

45. Sherwin, *No Longer Patient: Feminist Ethics and Health Care*, 89.

46. Sherwin, *No Longer Patient: Feminist Ethics and Health Care*, 13.

47. "My argument against oppression is a principled one, resting on a conception of justice that is defined in terms of its opposition to oppression." Sherwin, *No Longer Patient: Feminist Ethics and Health Care*, 82.

48. Sherwin, *No Longer Patient: Feminist Ethics and Health Care*, 32. Rosemarie Tong takes this "eclectic politics" as a characteristic feature of feminist bioethics, thus suggesting that all feminist approaches may be limited in a similar way. See Rosemarie Tong, *Feminist Approaches to Bioethics: Theoretical Reflections and Practical Applications* (Boulder, Colo.: Westview Press, 1997), 94.

49. H. Tristram Engelhardt, *The Foundations of Bioethics* (New York: Oxford University Press, 1996), 7.

50. Engelhardt, *The Foundations of Bioethics*, 7.

51. See Engelhardt, *The Foundations of Bioethics*, 94, n. 81.

52. Engelhardt, *The Foundations of Bioethics*, Ch. 2.

53. Engelhardt, *The Foundations of Bioethics*, 72.

54. Engelhardt, *The Foundations of Bioethics*, Ch. 4.

55. Jonsen, *The Birth of Bioethics*, 331.

56. John Arras, "A Taxonomy of Theoretical Work in Bioethics: Supplement to Theory and Bioethics," in *The Stanford Encyclopedia of Philosophy*, ed. Edward N. Zalta (2020). https://plato.stanford.edu/archives/fall2020/entries/theory-bioethics/supplement.html.

57. Beauchamp and Childress, *Principles of Biomedical Ethics*, 7th ed., 264.

58. Lewis Vaughn, *Bioethics: Principles, Issues, and Cases*, 3rd ed. (New York: Oxford University Press, 2017). At the date of writing, the 4th edition was the best-selling anthology in the "Medical Ethics" category on Amazon.

59. Rawls's theory of justice as fairness is often considered as a political theory, perhaps because Rawls calls it a theory of "justice," and because Rawls clearly expected that it could give normative guidance to governments. Rawls takes the theory primarily as a theory about justice, however, not a theory of government; on his view, justice is the "first virtue of social institutions," and the theory is designed for application to the "basic structure," by which he means the operation of the "political constitution and the principal economic and social arrangements." Rawls, *A Theory of Justice*, 7. So it is not clear in that work whether he recognizes any basic moral distinction between the norms governing the state and those governing other institutions of civil society, such as "competitive markets. . . . and the monogamous family." Rawls does seem to have come to appreciate a distinction to some extent in *Political Liberalism*, where he notes the distinctively coercive nature of the state. John Rawls, *Political Liberalism* (New York: Columbia University Press, 2005), 135–36; 216.

60. For example, see Bonnie Steinbock, John Arras, and Alex John London, *Ethical Issues in Modern Medicine*, 6th ed. (Boston: McGraw-Hill, 2003); Ronald Munson, *Intervention and Reflection: Basic Issues in Bioethics*, 8th ed. (Boston, MA: Wadsworth, Cengage Learning, 2008); David DeGrazia, Thomas A. Mappes, and Jeffrey Brand-Ballard, *Biomedical Ethics* (New York: McGraw-Hill Higher Education, 2011).

61. Vaughn, *Bioethics: Principles, Issues, and Cases*, 3rd ed., 7.

62. For example, see Alastair V. Campbell, *Bioethics: The Basics* (Milton Park, Abingdon, Oxon: Routledge, 2013).

63. Barry R. Furrow et al., *Bioethics: Health Care Law and Ethics*, 8th ed. (St. Paul, MN: West Academic Publishing, 2018).

64. See the discussion in Furrow et al., *Bioethics: Health Care Law and Ethics*, 8th ed., 28–30.

65. Janet L. Dolgin and Lois L. Shepherd, *Bioethics and the Law* (New York: Aspen Publishers, 2009), 13.

66. George J. Annas, *Standard of Care: The Law of American Bioethics* (New York: Oxford University Press, 1993); Barry R. Schaller, *Understanding Bioethics and the Law: The Promises and Perils of the Brave New World of Biotechnology* (Westport, Conn.: Praeger, 2008), x.

67. Bethany Spielman, *Bioethics in Law* (Totowa, N.J.: Humana Press, 2007).

68. Kenneth Veitch, *The Jurisdiction of Medical Law* (Burlington, VT: Ashgate, 2007).

69. Jerry Menikoff, *Law and Bioethics: An Introduction* (Washington, D.C.: Georgetown University Press, 2001), 1.

70. Arthur B. LaFrance, *Bioethics: Health Care, Human Rights, and the Law*, 2nd ed. (Newark, NJ: Matthew Bender, 2006); Marsha Garrison and Carl Schneider, *The Law of Bioethics: Individual Autonomy and Social Regulation*, 2nd ed., (St. Paul, MN: Thomson/West, 2009).

71. For example, see Norman Daniels, *Just Health Care* (New York: Cambridge University Press, 1985); Ezekiel J. Emanuel, *The Ends of Human Life: Medical Ethics in a Liberal Polity* (Cambridge, MA: Harvard University Press, 1991); Norman Daniels, *Just Health: Meeting Health Needs Fairly* (New York: Cambridge University Press, 2008).

72. This topic has obvious political aspects, which helps to explain the appearance of political theory here. Even so, political theory is not the focus of this literature; rather, it has tended to focus on whether bioethicists have "moral expertise" and if so, in what sense. See D. Robert MacDougall, "Liberalism, Authority, and Bioethics Commissions," *Theoretical Medicine and Bioethics* 34, no. 6 (2013).

Chapter 3

Bioethicists on Kant and the Legalization of Organ Markets

In order to illustrate more fully the tools and methods that characterize the contemporary bioethics approach to health law and policy, it will be helpful to give a detailed description of the literature applying Kantian philosophy to the question about whether organ sales or markets should be legalized. The prominence of Kantian philosophy in the literature on organ markets is a consequence in part of the specific comments Kant made about the moral permissibility of organ sales in his various moral works. This literature is robust and well-developed, and it explores a host of issues relevant to determining the relevance of Kant's arguments to the legalization of organ sales. However, despite the rich detail of this literature, which treats various questions in metaphysics, logic, and normative ethics, the vast majority of authors focus only on whether there is a primary moral duty not to sell organs. Very few address the question about what makes governments good, legitimate, or just. This oversight is shared by both those supporting the prohibition of organ sales and their critics. In other words, normative political philosophy barely features in this literature, despite its overt legal orientation. The description of this literature will conclude my empirical case that bioethics has neglected essential moral questions necessary for justifying law and policy, and clear the ground for the remaining discussion about the significance of this oversight.

I will begin with a brief explanation of Kant's moral philosophy. Then we will move to consider Kant's argument for his claim that selling organs is immoral. The bulk of the chapter, however, will be dedicated to showing that the authors discussing Kant's argument against organ-selling have widely assumed that if Kant is correct that organ-selling is immoral, then this would be an important reason for legally prohibiting it. In itself, their assumption is not surprising: as I explained in chapter 1, their assumption is widely shared in bioethics. In the following chapter (chapter 4), I will explain a significant problem with this assumption: Kantian moral philosophy itself does not support it.

UNDERSTANDING KANTIAN MORAL PHILOSOPHY

At least some understanding of Kantian moral philosophy will be important for understanding the arguments of the remainder of the book, particularly this chapter and the next.

Kant's earliest major work on moral philosophy is the *Groundwork for the Metaphysics of Morals*. It is still widely read in undergraduate ethics classes, and it is the work with which the majority of bioethics commentators are most familiar. Although Kant produced several more works on moral philosophy later in his career, the *Groundwork* is important because it outlines the fundamentals of his approach to practical philosophy, which his later works build on (as is evident from the term "groundwork" in the title).

Kant's philosophical project as a whole—his "critical" philosophy—can be best understood as a systematically developed account of the nature and limitations of reason. In his monumental *Critique of Pure Reason*, Kant outlines the nature and limits of theoretical reason, which is essentially the capacity of reason to determine *what is true*. But in the *Groundwork* he addresses questions related to practical reason, which is the capacity of reason to determine *what to do*. According to Kant, reason itself has various implications for what we should do. For example, if I set "arriving at work in the morning" as my end, reason demands that I take the necessary actions for achieving this end. In other words I must adjust my use of means such that they can accomplish my ends. To say that it is my end to go to work, but then fail to select means capable of accomplishing this, is to involve myself in a *contradiction* of practical reason: I both will and do not will, simultaneously, to accomplish my goal of arriving at work. The imperative here is what Kant calls a mere "hypothetical imperative," however, because it derives its force entirely from the fact that I have chosen arriving at work as my particular end: *if* my end is to go to work, *then* I must select means capable of achieving this end. If going to work is not my end, then reason does not require me to select any particular means with respect to that end.

Kant argues in the *Groundwork* that there are certain restrictions on the use of practical reason that are required by the capacity for reason itself, and are not dependent on the particular ends that people set for themselves. Kant says that these restrictions are prescribed by a *Categorical Imperative* of reason: "categorical" because it applies unconditionally, that is, without reference to the goals, interests, preferences, or other features of the individual agent. This Categorical Imperative prescribes the set of our moral duties, that is, the set of requirements imposed on all reasoning beings because they are imposed by reason itself. Because the Categorical Imperative is derived from the capacity for reason itself, to violate the Categorical Imperative at any time is to commit a "contradiction in practical reason"—that is, to violate the most basic rules governing the use of reason in our actions.

Instead of offering a single statement of the Categorical Imperative, Kant offers three "formulations" of it. He claims they all amount to the same thing, although each may be more or less helpful for determining the morality of our actions under different circumstances. Kant offers arguments for each, to show that they are objectively required by reason itself, and so can be considered universal and, consequently, morally binding. But the details of these arguments, while important, don't concern us here.[1] The three formulations of the Categorical Imperative, presented by Kant, are:

> Formula of Universal Law: Act only in accordance with that maxim through which you can at the same time will that it become a universal law.[2]

> Formula of Humanity: So act that you use humanity, whether in your own person or in the person of any other, always at the same time as an end, never merely as a means.[3]

> Formula of Autonomy: The idea of the will of every rational being as a will giving universal law.[4]

Kant uses these formulations to show how various actions, premised on underlying "maxims" (or subjective principles or reasons), can involve persons in internal contradictions, or put reason in contradiction with itself. For example, Kant explains that a person who intentionally lies in order to obtain some benefit for himself commits a contradiction in practical reason, insofar as he wills both that persons lie (as he is lying in this case), and that persons generally tell the truth (which practice is what makes the success of the lie possible), simultaneously.[5] The basic nature of the inconsistency can best be seen by looking at the first formulation, the Formula of Universal Law: the liar acts on a maxim (or principle) that he cannot will that everyone act on, universally. He wills the principle, "when I want to obtain some benefit I will lie," both as sufficient reason for action (when he applies it to his own case), and not as sufficient reason for action (when he applies it to people in general). Similarly, we can see that the Formula of Humanity also rules out the possibility of a lie: when the liar lies to obtain some benefit from someone else, he necessarily treats that person "merely as a means." Insofar as he conceives the lie as necessary for obtaining the benefit, the liar anticipates that it is not the other person's end to let him have it; by lying to her, he uses her as a mere means by making her believe something untrue so that her subsequent actions (giving him the thing he wants) will be instrumental to ends that she does not share. Lying is thus shown to involve a contradiction in practical reason, and as such to be immoral.

Kant derives a multitude of implications from these principles, including various implications for how we treat our bodies. One implication of the Categorical Imperative, says Kant, is that it strictly prohibits selling organs.

KANT ON ORGAN SALES

Kant's position on the morality of organ sales is well known, and the relevant texts are widely cited. In sum, Kant holds that persons may not maim, dismember, or otherwise permanently alter their bodies for any purpose other than to save their own lives. For example, Kant says persons are not permitted to sell limbs, even if they are "offered ten thousand thalers for a single finger."[6] Selling a tooth is wrong,[7] even if done to help someone in need of replacing "decayed dentition."[8] Even giving away a tooth is a way of "partially murdering oneself."[9] A man cannot have himself castrated to make it possible to earn a living as a singer.[10] Cutting one's hair is not a crime, since hair is not an integral organ, but cutting it to sell it is not "altogether free of blame."[11] Amputating a diseased limb to save one's own life, however, is permissible.[12]

Although Kant is abundantly clear about whether organ sales are permissible, his arguments showing why such sales are morally prohibited, regrettably, are not. Some of the quotations above are found in student notes from lectures given before his major works on morality were written, and are tied to principles or explanations that Kant later changed or abandoned. Moreover, in Kant's only discussion of organ sales in his major moral works, he condemns organ sales but does not explain in detail why such sales violate any formulation of the Categorical Imperative. This discussion occurs in the *Doctrine of Virtue* where Kant says that to "maim" oneself or "deprive oneself of an integral organ" (for example, to "sell a tooth") is to commit partial suicide.[13] Since Kant argues (both in this passage and elsewhere[14]) that suicide is wrong because it violates the Categorical Imperative, it seems natural to assume that Kant intends to condemn self-mutilation on the grounds that it violates the Categorical Imperative in the same way that suicide does. But the reasons for thinking suicide to be immoral on Kantian grounds, and the reasons for thinking that self-mutilation is a form of partial suicide, are themselves open to debate.

KANTIAN ARGUMENTS FOR LEGAL PROHIBITION

Perhaps because of the complexity and obscurity of Kant's arguments, bioethicists have offered diverse explanations about the implications of Kantian principles for prohibitions against organ sales. In trying to understand the Kantian argument, commentators have generally turned either to the Formula of Humanity or the idea of human dignity to explain the Kantian moral objection to organ sales. The remainder of this chapter will explore the way that these arguments have featured in the debate about legal prohibitions against organ sales, followed by the critical response to these arguments that has developed in the bioethics literature.

Before beginning, note that the following discussion aims at comprehensiveness. Specifically, I have tried to incorporate all the sources making substantive use of Kantian philosophy to ground normative conclusions about laws and policies governing organ sales.[15] The taxonomy of arguments I provide in this chapter is, similarly, intended to reflect all the major arguments that have been put forth in this debate in the bioethics literature as well. Treating this literature comprehensively is important because it will allow us to see the detail and rigor of the bioethics literature applying Kantian philosophy to the issue of organ sales, but also to see the almost complete absence of normative political philosophy in this literature.

Formula of Humanity

As we saw, Kant's Formula of Humanity requires using humanity always as an end and never merely as a means. Treating others as a mere means is problematic, essentially, because it treats them in a way that we cannot will persons to be treated as a general rule. Kant argues that when we act on our own ends, we treat those ends as intrinsically valuable. But when we treat others as a mere means, we treat their ends as though they are valuable only instrumentally toward our own. Insofar as we treat them as mere means to our ends, we assign an importance to their ends that we are not willing to assign to human ends in general, and thus commit a contradiction in practical reason.

What does it mean, to refrain from treating others as a mere means? One way of understanding the Kantian prohibition here is to interpret it as a requirement to avoid treating persons merely as any of the things that are typically used to meet our interests. Consequently, Kant explicitly rejects uses of persons that are reminiscent of the ways in which persons use tools, objects, possessions, and tradable commodities.

Commentators who support prohibitions of organ sales have subsequently drawn on these metaphors to explain the wrongfulness of organ sales. Leon

Kass, for example, cites Kant's argument that persons who sell kidneys "dispose" of themselves, much as one does an object or possession, thus degrading the humanity in their person.[16] Mario Morelli finds that commercial sales "instrumentalize" and "objectify" persons in ways that donations do not.[17] However, for Morelli it is ultimately the importance of maintaining important values, like humanity, dignity, and the equal worth of all, that justifies legal prohibitions against sales.

While these authors suggest that all organ sales treat someone as a mere means, Stephen Munzer finds that only some sales treat persons as mere means.[18] Munzer argues that if sales are done for mere compensation, then they obviously seem to treat persons as commodities or possessions, and so as mere means. However, sales to fulfill a duty of beneficence seem to treat persons as ends. Munzer reasons that, since Kant did not know that organ transplants would one day be capable of saving lives, he could not consider whether removing organs might in such cases effectively treat persons as ends. Assuming that Kant would agree that removing organs is permissible in cases where it saves lives, he might even approve of some sales: there is no reason, for example, why a person could not sell an organ and use the proceeds to care for a sick loved one. According to Munzer, the Formula of Humanity thus only prohibits sales in *some* cases.[19]

A second strand of argument developed from the Formula of Humanity proceeds along very different lines. Although Ronald Green is also concerned about treating other persons as mere means, he argues that Kant fails to show that there is anything inherently wrong with organ sales. He concludes that Kant's claims about the immorality of such sales are likely little more than "refined prejudices" inherited from his Christian background.[20] However, Green offers a different reading of the Formula of Humanity that nevertheless may have important consequences for markets in organs. Kant's Formula of Humanity requires treating others as ends in themselves, and so we must impartially consider the consequences of "open and legal markets" in organs for all others. According to Green, wealthy Westerners may suffer no ill consequences from such markets. The global poor however are relatively more likely to suffer and less likely to benefit from such a market, so markets in organs risk treating them as mere means.

Human Dignity

Kant's discussion of human dignity occurs in the *Groundwork,* in connection with his explanation of the third formulation of the Categorical Imperative, the Formula of Autonomy. Kant argues there that humanity's capacity to give laws to itself is what endows humanity with a "dignity above all price."[21]

The argument from dignity is closely connected to the argument from humanity. We have already noted that treating others as mere means treats them in a way that is necessarily incompatible with the way in which we could will to be treated, because it is not possible for us to will that our own ends be subservient to the ends of others. Consequently, we must treat their ends—and so, them—as intrinsically valuable, in the same way we treat our own ends and thus, ourselves. If persons are intrinsically valuable, then we cannot place a price on them: they are ends in themselves, not capable of being bought or sold for some other purpose. They possess a dignity above all price.

We can distinguish the idea of a "dignity above all price" from the idea of being an end in oneself in the following way. As noted above, Kant uses a variety of glosses for "means," including instruments, things, and objects. This formulation is consequently best suited to qualitative interpretations: persons must be treated as persons, and not as any other kind of entity. The idea of human dignity, however, has to do with the worth attached to humanity, and thus suggests a quantitative interpretation: the dignity of humanity supersedes any price that might be put on it.

It is worth pointing out that Kant never explicitly attributed dignity to the human body or any of its parts. However, since Kant claims that everything in the kingdom of ends has either a "price or a dignity,"[22] and seems to express that body parts should not have a price,[23] it seems unproblematic to infer that for Kant, bodies and body parts must have a dignity as well. Organ sales seem to violate the Kantian precept, then, primarily because they associate an *actual price* with a person or part thereof.

Several commentators have consequently concluded that markets in organs are prohibited by Kant's account of the dignity of humanity. Cynthia Cohen argues that Kantian dignity demonstrates that the "human community should not permit individuals to give over integral parts of their bodies for money."[24] Gerrand,[25] Powers,[26] and Alpinar-Şencan[27] also argue that Kant would prohibit markets in organs but understand the Kantian argument from dignity as prohibiting not only sales but also donations (for reasons we shall discuss later in this chapter).

Some authors have sought to make use of the Kantian idea of dignity without thinking that dignity need apply to body parts in the same way that it applies to persons as a whole. For these authors, putting a price on a body as a whole would offend dignity, but putting a price on a part may or may not. Stephen Munzer argues that body parts fall diversely onto a "gradient" of dignity, where the dignity of the body part is determined by how "integral" the organ is to the functioning of a human body, or alternatively, how intimately associated the organ is with that body.[28] On Munzer's view, selling an organ may offend dignity if the seller sells for reasons that are not strong enough relative to the dignity of the organ being sold. Such a sale does not actually reduce the dignity of the organ but does "insult" or "demean" its dignity. Rom Harré, likewise, argues that body parts attain their "value" from different sources.[29] Some parts, like the heart or lungs, gain their value from their necessity for sustaining life; sale of these is thus prohibited. Other parts, like kidneys, gain their value primarily from their close relationship to a human body. Organs like kidneys can be compared to items like a '33 Bugati or an art masterpiece: the value attached to them prohibits their destruction or other undignified uses but does not necessarily prohibit buying or selling them, assuming that the seller intends to treat the purchased item with the appropriate kind of respect.

Finally, some authors have argued that, even if organ sales do not inherently violate human dignity, they may nevertheless be objectionable on Kantian grounds in some circumstances insofar as they diminish the *sense* of dignity or equality possessed by various persons. To assess whether real markets actually offend against dignity in this way, Munzer embarks on a lengthy casuistical analysis, assessing whether sales might harm the "sense" of dignity of various parties in various circumstances. Sales might affect the sense of dignity of the sellers differently from the sense of dignity of the buyers, and these will yet be different from the effects on the sense of dignity of "intermediaries" (like health care workers) and those of uninvolved third parties. Determining whether a sale or market poses a "risk to dignity," then, takes "analytical skill and empirical information." But ultimately, such a complex analysis can help us to assess the overall acceptability of the market. Such markets are "morally objectionable" if their "operation offends the dignity of enough participants in the market."

Kerstein, similarly, after rejecting a variety of Kantian arguments thought to show why sales are impermissible, notes that Kant requires acting in ways that do not seem to express disrespect for the worth or dignity of other persons.[30] Kerstein notes that a kidney sale may tend to "encourage or promote the notion" that persons themselves—most likely the poor, who already have a lower social status—are for sale. In cases where sales seem to express that poor persons themselves are for sale, and so are not equal in dignity and worth to others, the sales are wrong. However, whether organ sales express this idea will vary significantly according to cultural and social ideas about the equality of persons, as well as to overall social stratification.

PROBLEMS WITH KANTIAN ARGUMENTS FOR LEGAL PROHIBITIONS

Regardless of whether one grounds Kantian prohibitions in the argument from humanity or from dignity, several serious problems or obstacles remain for those who would utilize Kant's moral philosophy in contemporary debates about organ sales. Critics and proponents of organ markets alike have noticed these problems, and the resulting debate is a testament to the overall robustness of the literature on this topic. However, with few exceptions, critics have not engaged in discussion about the morality of governmental intervention in organ sales. Instead, critics have engaged in this debate by questioning either the correctness of Kant's moral theory or the plausibility of the conclusions he drew from it. In so doing, they reinforce the assumption that the moral status of particular actions, rather than the moral status of the laws or activities of governments that regulate them, are the most important factor in determining the legal status of those actions.

The Failure of Kantian Moral Theory

The most general problem with applying Kant's moral philosophy to contemporary debates is related to the failure of Kantian moral theory itself. There are at least two ways of presenting this problem.

Failure of Comprehensive Doctrines in General

First, some point out that there are difficulties with justifying laws on Kantian grounds because Kant—like other moral theorists before and after him—was not successful in conclusively demonstrating his moral theory. The problem, according to Engelhardt, is that contemporary "ethical" justifications for laws prohibiting organ sales must proceed from some canonical secular morality, but no canonical secular morality can be conclusively demonstrated by reason. While Kant claimed to have demonstrated such a canonical secular morality, he had to presuppose the existence of God and of immortality just to make plausible his most basic claim that the right has priority over the good.[31] Contemporary bioethicists employing Kant to defend prohibitions against kidney sales not only overlook these controversial assumptions, but also selectively endorse the implications that Kant himself claimed follow from his principles. For example, they endorse his view that human dignity rules out the permissibility of selling organs, while neglecting to mention that Kant also thought that human dignity rules out the permissibility of masturbation.[32] Engelhardt argues that, because legal prohibitions are coercive and can have serious effects on individual welfare, any justification short of rational necessitation seems insufficient. Coercive prohibitions justified by reference to Kantian philosophy are, effectively, unjustifiable instances of imposing one's views on nonconsenting, peaceable, and innocent others.[33]

Gill and Sade (in a response to the essays by Cohen and Morelli mentioned earlier) make a similar point.[34] Gill and Sade point out that even if Kant's theories of autonomy and human dignity were fundamentally correct, Kant's theory is far too demanding to be the basis for laws in a pluralistic society. In fact, the well-established legal doctrine of informed consent is based on the idea that no thick moral notions should serve as the basis for coercive laws. Instead, laws should be based on a "thin" and "noninterference" conception of autonomy. If individual self-determination can be trumped by "robust" Kantian notions of autonomy in cases concerning the sale of organs, presumably it can be trumped by Kantian autonomy in clinical decision making as well. This would mean that patients would not be permitted to make decisions that were not sufficiently well-motivated or were not based on a full sense of the worth of humanity, which would overturn the decades-long legal stance that patients have a right to refuse treatment for any reason by withholding informed consent. For Engelhardt and Gill and Sade, then, the problems with enforcing Kantian views are not tied to the failure of Kant's views specifically; perhaps no view can be conclusively demonstrated. The problem is rather with enforcing *any* view that is reasonably disputed.

Failure of Kant's View in Particular

A second way in which the Kantian arguments for prohibition have been countered is by calling into question Kant's success in particular. Was Kant successful in demonstrating his various formulations of the Categorical Imperative? According to Thomas J. Bole III, the answer is a qualified "no."[35] Kant was successful in demonstrating that the condition for moral responsibility is freedom. If persons are to be held morally responsible for their actions, we must consider them—and they must actually be—free of coercive factors. The Formula of Humanity, which prohibits non-consensual interference with others on the grounds that such interference treats them as mere means, effectively protects the freedom necessary for moral responsibility. Consequently, Bole argues that Kant establishes that persons must be treated as ends in themselves—in the sense of not being used without consent—since this is a condition for the possibility of morality. According to Bole, Kant successfully shows that respecting others as ends in themselves functions as a side-constraint on what it is possible to do to them.

However, Bole argues that Kant's more ambitious project—the positive project that requires us to seek the happiness of others and never to will the destruction of the body—is an unequivocal failure. Showing that we may not violate the conditions of another's freedom is not the same as showing that we have a positive responsibility to contribute to it. Bole considers the consequences of this failure for Congress's criminalization of organ sales. Far from underwriting this law, Bole argues that Kant actually shows why such a law is immoral. Insofar as persons consent to sell their organs, it cannot even be shown that they treat themselves as a mere means. For if they give their consent, the sale of the organ has their approval and thus the sale is one of their ends. Consequently, third parties who would interfere in such consensual market exchanges in the name of upholding Kant's content-full vision of what it means to respect persons as ends would actually be *undermining* the condition of the freedom of the transacting parties, and thus would be acting immorally.

Problems with Application

The great bulk of criticism aimed at Kantian prohibitions on kidney sales has focused, however, not on the success of Kantian moral theory, but rather on the plausibility of applying Kant's moral theory to legal prohibitions against organ sales in the way that proponents of prohibitions do.

The Fallacy of Division

Perhaps the most frequently discussed problem with Kant's arguments relates to metaphysical assumptions Kant employs in his arguments against selling organs. As we pointed out earlier, Kant draws a sharp distinction between persons and all other things. Persons are ends in themselves, possessed of a dignity above all price; nothing else has these distinctions. For example, elsewhere in his writings Kant distinguishes sharply between "persons and property."[36] Kant assumes that the special status accorded to persons has implications for how they may treat their bodies, but this seems problematic because it is not entirely clear why moral conclusions about persons apply to their body parts.

Rom Harré was perhaps the first to discuss this problem.[37] Stephen Munzer, however, develops the problem more thoroughly. The main problem with Kant's actual argument, says Munzer, is that it is simply "not enough to assert that it is 'impossible to be a person and a thing.'"[38] Why couldn't our bodies be *both* persons and things? Moreover, even if Kant is right to say that persons and things are nonoverlapping metaphysical categories, it isn't at all clear why our body parts would fall into the former category rather than the latter. Kant assumes that if the body has a special metaphysical status as a "person," then this metaphysical status must apply to each component part of the body as well. But, says Munzer, this is the "fallacy of division," because one cannot draw a conclusion about the nature of the part directly from the nature of the whole. My car may be green, but it does not follow that the exhaust pipe is green. But Kant seems to assume, in all cases where he draws implications for treatment of body parts from his moral principles, that the parts will contain the properties of the whole.

Munzer considers several possible Kantian responses to the "fallacy of division" problem. Two are important. First, we might stipulate that persons simply are constituted by their body parts. Kant seems to have done just that.[39] If persons are constituted of bodies (and presumably, body parts) by definition, then this could explain why treating the body (or one of its parts) in some way is the same as treating the humanity in the person in that way. However, Kant's definition of a person is not widely accepted, and worse, it seems to rely on Kant's infamous phenomenal/noumenal distinction, which is complicated and widely rejected.[40]

Second, the Kantian argument could rely exclusively on the moral status of whole persons, rather than on the moral status of their parts.[41] This would entail understanding vital body parts (such as lungs and hearts) as constitutive of persons because these are necessary for survival of the whole person; but non-vital parts (such as fingers, teeth, or extra kidneys), as simply property or things. However, this position is obviously at odds with Kant's own conclusions. So, for Munzer, this Kantian argument either relies on a dubious metaphysics or fails to establish the conclusion with respect to (at least non-vital) body parts.

Several authors have tried to defend Kant against the "fallacy of division" argument. Nicole Gerrand concedes that Munzer is essentially correct when he claims that Kant's view about human bodies relies on his metaphysics, but she thinks Munzer overrates the problems with Kant's metaphysics.[42] Kant's view is simply that bodies constitute persons. Since body parts constitute the body, they also constitute the person. So to treat a body part as a thing is also to treat the person as a thing. Cynthia Cohen responds to the problem in a similar way: according to Cohen, Kant regards kidneys as *integral* organs which means they "just are the person," and so cannot be sold without thereby seeming to "impugn" human dignity.[43]

But these authors miss the point here: what is needed is an explanation about *why* Kant was justified in identifying body parts, even teeth, with the person herself; and these authors merely reiterate Kant's stipulation that the body *is* the person.

Jean-Christophe Merle engages in a meticulous reading of Kant and finds that Kant divides the body into three kinds of parts: vital organs, integral organs, and mere accumulations.[44] Vital organs are those organs necessary for survival; integral organs are integrated into functioning systems of the body and cannot be replenished (but are not strictly necessary for survival);

and mere accumulations are parts like skin, hair, and bone marrow that can be replenished. On Merle's reading of Kant, dismemberment involving either vital or integral organs is wrong, but for different reasons. Dismemberment of vital organs is wrong because it is essentially suicide; vital organs are organs necessary for continued life. Munzer is correct to think that we cannot have "property" in vital organs, according to Merle, since disposing of these organs leads to the death of the agent. However, dismemberment involving "integral" but not "vital" organs is wrong for a different reason altogether. Such dismemberments would reduce an individual's "freedom of choice," says Merle, referring to a concept from Kant's *Doctrine of Right*. Thus if Kant's prohibition against the sale of integral organs does not rely on the same rationale as the prohibition against the sale of vital organs, then he does not need to assume that the parts will possess the same properties as the whole, and so there is no fallacy of division.[45]

Alpinar-Sencan responds to arguments (such as Merle's) that try to distinguish between different parts of the body by explaining why this interpretation of Kant is not one he has left open to us. Essentially, Alpinar-Sencan argues that Kant does not divide the body into a hierarchy of parts.[46] On her reading, Kant does not think either that some body parts are more central to our identity than others, nor that the moral status of a body part depends on the role it plays in normal human function. If the body "constitutes" the person, then each part derives its overall status from the status of the person as a whole.

Alpinar-Sencan suggests—like Gerrand—that Kant's arguments apply to separating *any* body part from the person. While Alpinar-Sencan and Gerrand are probably correct in their reading of Kant, and thus effectively show why Merle's attempt to save Kant fails, neither answers the challenge Munzer presents in the fallacy of division argument. Kant's prohibition against selling any nonessential organs such as an extra kidney depends on the idea that selling the parts is morally equivalent to selling the whole. Insofar as Kant's view here relies on a mere stipulation, the view seems arbitrary. Insofar as it depends on Kantian metaphysics, it seems problematic.

The Self-Preservation Exception

Beyond the metaphysical problems that accompany prohibitions grounded in Kantian theory, a second problem is related to Kant's admission that there are some exceptions to the general prohibition against self-mutilation. Namely, Kant comments that a "diseased limb" may be removed if it is necessary to save a life. And, as James Stacey Taylor notes, Kant also suggests that circumcision might be permissible even when there is no disease.[47] Kant relates a story he has heard about a Frenchman who was forced to accept circumcision on pain of death when visiting Mecca to observe "Mohammedan ceremonies." Why should I not accept circumcision, says Kant, "particularly if I thereby save my life?"[48]

Taylor and others have made much of the fact that Kant allows this exception to the general rule.[49] If Kant allows this exception, it might seem to create latitude not only for self-mutilation but even for sales in some circumstances. As Chadwick notes, it is conceivable that a person might sell an organ because he fears death at the hands of loan sharks to whom he owes money.[50] And, if a person can sell an organ to save his or her own life, it might also seem plausible that a person could sell an organ to save the life of someone else. Since the general rationale for kidney sales is that they will save lives, and since certainly some sellers can be anticipated to sell for this reason, the self-preservation exception might seem to justify a kidney market all by itself.

Sales but Not Donations?

A third problem with arguments grounding prohibitions in Kantian theory follows from the fact that the Kantian arguments suggest *all* instances of self-mutilation are morally impermissible (except in cases of self-preservation). In other words, if the Kantian arguments succeed, then—as Kant himself mentions[51]—both sales *and* donations are impermissible. This only poses a problem for those commentators who wish to deploy Kantian arguments against sales while permitting a system of organ donations. This is a major problem for most of those employing Kant to argue against organ markets, however, since most of these authors do wish to preserve a system allowing for kidney donations.

Several commentators who oppose sales have proposed Kantian reasons for permitting donations. These authors have pointed to the fact that Kant did not know about the lifesaving potential of kidney transplants. Leon Kass argues that donations, but not sales, can be justified by the goods they obtain (namely, preserving life).[52] Stephen Munzer mentions the "ill-considered" passage in which Kant forbids donating a tooth: surely, he comments, if Kant had known about the lifesaving potential of kidney transplants, he would have supported donations.[53] Cynthia Cohen argues that, although Kant would have prohibited organ sales, if he had known about transplantation he would have permitted donations (so long as they do not "destroy integrity" by killing or seriously damaging the donor) because donations promote "altruism and solidarity with other human beings."[54] Morelli, similarly, explains that the major difference between donations and sales is that donations can be done for reasons of beneficence, such as saving a life, while sales always treat persons as mere means.[55] And Heubel and Biller-Andorno argue that Kant gives arguments suggesting organ donation may be permissible in cases where it is not done from "self-love,"[56] but that he would hold that organ sales are always immoral "irrespective of the circumstances," because they put a price on something with dignity, and thus degrade it.[57]

Although many would like Kant to support something like the current scheme of prohibiting sales but permitting donations, it is unlikely Kant can support this. There are several reasons—beyond his explicit condemnation of organ donations—for believing that Kant sees no principled distinction between donations and sales. First is the fact, already noted, that Kant objects to all instances of self-mutilation, not just those involving sales. Second, the fact that something is not sold does not mean it has no price, and so doesn't guarantee that it respects human dignity. For Kant, a thing has a "price" when it is treated as having a value in some way relative to "interests and needs."[58] Presumably, then, organ donations—which occur precisely because they are of value to the interests and needs of the recipient—are also forbidden. Third, Kant mentions that something has a price if it can be exchanged for something else as its equivalent, that is if it is treated as "interchangeable" with other things like it.[59] A donated organ, of course, is desirable precisely because it can serve as a replacement to a malfunctioning organ, and any particular donated organ is interchangeable with other similar organs also in the donor pool. In this way, donated organs are treated as fungible in a way that persons themselves are not. It is for these reasons that the authors reading Kant most closely have rejected the idea that Kant could support donations but not sales.[60]

Even though many of Kant's examples of self-mutilation mention money, Kant is actually concerned with any action that permanently destroys or impairs the human body at all.[61] This reading of Kant is required by the fact that he calls the various forms of self-mutilation "partial self-murder": they permanently destroy part of the self. It also helps explain why Kant treats self-mutilation as similar in kind to self-induced temporary incapacitation (probably imagining the influence of either alcohol or opiates).[62] Kant classifies both mutilation and self-induced incapacitation as violations of a person's duty to "himself as an animal being." Temporary incapacitation impairs the self, but has little to do with commodification or the exchange of money. It is unlikely, then that Kant can successfully distinguish between sales and donations because his primary concern does not appear to be about money at all.

The fact that Kant would treat sales and donations in the same way probably represents the most significant obstacle for using Kant's moral philosophy to support a ban on kidney sales, at least among the obstacles recognized in the literature to this point. Kant's inability to distinguish between the two has convinced some authors to reject Kantian arguments on this issue altogether. Alpinar-Sencan, for example, argues that none of the Kantian arguments against organ sales are "compelling" because, insofar as they succeed in forbidding sales, they also succeed in forbidding donations.[63] Cècile Fabre also notes that insofar as Kantian objections suggest the impermissibility of organ donations, they seem to prove too much.[64]

Other authors, however, have been willing to bite the bullet on this. If Kantian moral principles prohibit live organ donation, then so much the worse for live organ donation. Both Thomas Powers[65] and JC Merle[66] seem to reach something like this conclusion. However, as both point out, donations and sales after death are another matter; after death the body can no longer be considered a "person" in the Kantian sense of a rational being. Consequently, donations should be permitted after death. Merle even argues that it might be a "duty of right" for persons to donate their organs after death.[67]

POLITICAL PHILOSOPHY IN THE DEBATE ABOUT KANTIAN PROHIBITIONS ON ORGAN SALES

Although nearly all authors discussing the various Kantian arguments have sought to resolve the legality question by appealing directly to primary moral rights and duties, a few have gone further by considering the question of secondary rights and duties, that is, the question about the ethics of intervening in such sales.[68] I count three authors who have made contributions in this direction; all are critics of prohibiting organ sales. First, Robert Taylor criticizes earlier authors, pointing out that they address whether markets will diminish Kantian autonomy without addressing whether persons may nevertheless have "self-ownership."[69] It is possible that such sales diminish autonomy but are also in some sense rightful because persons have self-ownership, such that interfering with these sales would be wrong.

Taylor's argument, like that of the proponents of legal prohibitions, depends on arguments from various formulations of the Categorical Imperative.[70] However, Taylor reaches very different conclusions about the implications of these arguments. According to Taylor, interference with persons' self-regarding choices violates the autonomy of rational persons because the interference treats them either paternalistically or, worse, as a mere means to an end. Taylor reasons that if third parties have a perfect and universal duty not to interfere with persons' bodies without their consent, then persons must have property rights in their bodies (Kant's claims to the contrary notwithstanding—these, Taylor argues, are based on Kant's misunderstanding of the meaning of property rights). And if persons have Kantian property rights in their bodies, then this justifies rights to transfer their body parts, although not necessarily to be compensated for the transfer.

Similarly, Dominic Wilkinson argues that even if we grant that selling organs violates human dignity, it does not follow that such sales should thereby be legally prohibited.[71] In fact, legal prohibition also violates human dignity because it treats persons as incapable of making their own choices, thus diminishing their dignity. Wilkinson points to one of Kant's early political writings to support his claim that Kant would have opposed paternalistic state interference with individuals, even when their choices are bad.[72]

And Bole, as we have seen, argues that the Formula of Humanity actually precludes the permissibility of *prohibitions* on organ sales: a person who sells an organ has this sale as one of their ends, and interference with another person's free pursuit of ends treats that person as a mere means.[73]

These authors are important outliers in this debate. They suggest a way forward, albeit incompletely, by focusing not on the primary moral duties of those selling their organs, but instead on the duties and rights of those who would interfere. This is an incipient form of political philosophy. These authors recognize that the most important question when considering prohibitions on organ sales is whether it is legitimate to interfere with such sales, and if so, on what grounds. Questions about the moral permissibility of sales are only relevant if we assume a certain kind of answer to the legitimacy question.

Despite the fact that this is a promising beginning to resolving problems about regulating the sale of organs, it is ultimately unsatisfactory for two reasons. First, although these authors focus on the ethics of intervening in organ sales rather than organ-selling itself, all three propose to answer the question about laws by appealing to Kant's theory of moral duties. They each argue some form of the idea that Kant's moral philosophy shows that it is immoral to intervene in organ sales. But this is problematic because, even if their arguments successfully show that it is normally impermissible for moral agents to intervene in organ sales, it is not at all clear that this conclusion should apply straightforwardly to *governments*. Governments do, and are reasonably expected to do, a whole host of things that would be immoral for ordinary agents to do. For example, governments collect taxes and put people in prison. If governments were bound by the same moral rules as ordinary citizens, then it would seem implausible that they would be permitted to do these things. As we shall see in chapter 4, the idea that governments are entitled to engage in such activities presents a difficult problem for Kantian ethics. I will argue in chapter 6 that Kant is only able to solve these problems by developing an account of political philosophy that does not depend directly on any of the formulations of the Categorical Imperative. The arguments of these authors are inconclusive, then, because showing that it is normally impermissible to intervene in organ sales does not yet show that government intervention is impermissible. For that, it seems we would need a theory of government.

Second, this approach is unsatisfactory because, even if it could answer questions about the legitimacy of interfering with organ sales, it leaves unanswered many of the important questions that remain about the regulation of organ sales. Suppose, for example, we assume with these authors that Kant shows both that organ sales are morally impermissible but that it is also morally impermissible to prohibit such sales. Nevertheless, governments must take a stance with respect to various issues involved in such exchanges, including whether it will enforce contracts for these immoral sales, whether it will collect sales taxes on them, and how it will regard the status of transplanted organs (Are they property? Or are they persons or parts thereof, and if so, which persons—the vendor or the recipient?). To answer such questions, we need a theory about what makes government just or legitimate or good, not just a single principle of morally permissible intervention. I will give an account about how Kant's theory of government provides a basis for answering some of these more complicated political questions in chapters 5, 6, and 7.

MORALITY AS THE BASIS FOR LEGAL PROHIBITIONS?

The vast majority of commentary addressing the relevance of Kantian philosophy to organ sales focuses on the plausibility of Kant's account of primary moral duties contained in the Categorical Imperative and on whether that account establishes the existence of a moral duty not to sell one's organs. Commentators in this debate almost universally assume that if it can be shown that there is a primary moral duty not to sell one's organs, then this would constitute a justification for legal prohibitions on such sales. They seem to assume that the overriding purpose of laws is to enforce morality. But this is an inference, since they never address this point explicitly, much less defend or explain it in light of general considerations about what makes government just or legitimate or good.

The fact that proponents of prohibitions do this might not suggest, by itself, that there is a problem with the bioethics literature. It is possible to imagine a literature in which bioethicists who rely on unstated premises of this type are routinely challenged to explain why they think governments should enforce our moral obligations. But as we have seen, critics have implicitly endorsed the unstated premises. They overwhelmingly challenge proponents of prohibitions by questioning whether Kant succeeds in demonstrating a primary moral duty not to sell one's organs, or on whether such a duty would apply to contemporary organ markets, and not by questioning the implicit theory of government underlying these accounts. Although it is widely accepted that just because something is immoral does not mean that it need be illegal, for some reason critics have generally refrained from making this point, and instead tried to establish that the Kantian arguments fail to establish the relevant moral duty.

Unlike the commentators on both sides of the contemporary literature, Kant himself did not assume that governments should enforce our moral obligations (at least, not *because* they are moral obligations). Ironically, the strongest (and likely the easiest) case that can be made against supposedly "Kantian" support for legal prohibitions comes from consideration of Kant's own writing about the distinction between legality and morality. In his political philosophy, Kant argues—rightly, as I shall explain in chapter 4—that moral principles of the type found in the Categorical Imperative, universally utilized by both proponents of prohibitions and their critics, are not a sufficient basis for laws at all.

However, perhaps it is because of the overall absence of attention to political philosophy that authors in this debate have not seen fit to utilize even Kant's own political philosophy when addressing the application of Kantian philosophy to organ sales. The general features of the debate surrounding the legality of organ sales are the strongest evidence I will present that bioethicists have neglected to make significant use of political philosophy, preferring instead to evaluate laws and policies by focusing on the primary moral duties that these target.

NOTES

1. For a good general introduction, see Allen W. Wood, "The Supreme Principle of Morality," in *The Cambridge Companion to Kant and Modern Philosophy*, ed. Paul Guyer (New York: Cambridge University Press, 2006).

2. Immanuel Kant, "Groundwork of the Metaphysics of Morals," in *Practical Philosophy*, ed. and trans. Mary J. Gregor, The Cambridge Edition of the Works of Immanuel Kant (New York: Cambridge University Press, 1996), 4:421. Excepting references to the *Doctrine of Right*, references to Kant's writings will be made by title only and will refer to the translation in this volume, unless otherwise noted. References to the *Doctrine of Right* are indicated by page numbers only, and refer to the edition found in Immanuel Kant, *The Metaphysics of Morals*, ed. Mary J. Gregor (New York: Cambridge University Press, 1996). All references to Kant's works use the Prussian Academy pagination.

3. *Groundwork*, 4:429.

4. *Groundwork*, 4:431.

5. *Groundwork*, 4:403.

6. Immanuel Kant, *Lectures on Ethics*, trans. Louis Infield (Indianapolis: Hackett Pub. Co., 1980), 124.

7. Kant, *Lectures on Ethics*, 165.

8. Immanuel Kant, *Lectures on Ethics*, ed. Peter Lauchlan Heath and J. B. Schneewind (New York: Cambridge University Press, 1997), 27:594.

9. *Doctrine of Virtue*, 6:423.

10. *Doctrine of Virtue* 6:423.
11. *Doctrine of Virtue* 6:423.
12. *Doctrine of Virtue* 6:423.
13. *Doctrine of Virtue* 6:423.
14. *Groundwork*, 4:421–22, 4:429.
15. Omitting only my own work on this topic. D. Robert MacDougall, "Sometimes Merely as a Means: Why Kantian Philosophy Requires the Legalization of Kidney Sales," *The Journal of Medicine and Philosophy* 44, no. 3 (2019).
16. Leon R Kass, "Organs for Sale? Propriety, Property, and the Price of Progress," *The Public Interest*, no. 107 (1993); Leon Kass, *Life, Liberty, and the Defense of Dignity: The Challenge for Bioethics*, 1st ed. (San Francisco: Encounter Books, 2002), 184–85.
17. Mario Morelli, "Commerce in Organs: A Kantian Critique," *Journal of Social Philosophy* 30, no. 2 (2004).
18. Stephen R Munzer, "Kant and Property Rights in Body Parts," *Canadian Journal of Law and Jurisprudence* 6 (1993).
19. In Munzer's wording, Kant's arguments can only show that we lack "property rights" in body parts in some cases. Munzer thinks that if moral sales are impermissible in some case, that means property rights to the body part are also lacking in that case.
20. Ronald M Green, "What Does It Mean to Use Someone as 'a Means Only': Rereading Kant," *Kennedy Institute of Ethics Journal* 11, no. 3 (2001).
21. *Groundwork*, 4:434–35.
22. *Groundwork*, 4:434.
23. Kant comments that a human being cannot sell his limbs for money, even were he offered "ten thousand thalers for a single finger." The clear implication is that the finger is worth more than any price that could be attached to it. Kant, *Lectures on Ethics*, 124.
24. Cynthia B. Cohen, "Selling Bits and Pieces of Humans to Make Babies: The Gift of the Magi Revisited," *The Journal of Medicine and Philosophy* 24, no. 3 (1999). See a similar argument in the later Cynthia B Cohen, "Public Policy and the Sale of Human Organs," *Kennedy Institute of Ethics Journal* 12, no. 1 (2002).
25. Nicole Gerrand, "The Misuse of Kant in the Debate About a Market for Human Body Parts," *Journal of Applied Philosophy* 16, no. 1 (1999).
26. Thomas M. Powers, "The Integrity of Body: Kantian Moral Constraints on the Physical Self," in *Persons and Their Bodies: Rights, Responsibilities, Relationships*, ed. Mark J. Cherry (Boston: Kluwer Academic, 1999).
27. Zümrüt Alpinar-Şencan, "Reconsidering Kantian Arguments against Organ Selling," *Medicine, Health Care and Philosophy* 19, no. 1 (2015).
28. Munzer suggests the violation of human dignity in his 1993 article, but the following discussion is taken from his more developed account in "An Uneasy Case against Property Rights in Body Parts," *Social Philosophy and Policy* 11, no. 2 (1994).
29. Rom Harré, "Bodily Obligations," *Cogito* 1, no. 3 (1987).
30. Samuel Kerstein, "Kantian Condemnation of Commerce in Organs," *Kennedy Institute of Ethics Journal* 19, no. 2 (2009). Kerstein also makes a very similar

argument in "Autonomy, Moral Constraints, and Markets in Kidneys," *Journal of Medicine and Philosophy* 34, no. 6 (2009).

31. H. T. Engelhardt, "The Injustice of Enforced Equal Access to Transplant Operations: Rethinking Reckless Claims of Fairness," *The Journal of Law, Medicine, & Ethics* 35, no. 2 (2007).

32. H. Tristram Engelhardt Jr., "The Body for Fun, Beneficence and Profit: A Variation on a Post-Modern Theme," in *Persons and Their Bodies: Rights, Responsibilities, Relationships*, ed. Mark J. Cherry (Dordrecht; Boston: Kluwer Academic, 1999).

33. H. T. Engelhardt, "The Injustice of Enforced Equal Access to Transplant Operations: Rethinking Reckless Claims of Fairness," *The Journal of Law, Medicine, & Ethics* 35, no. 2 (2007).

34. Michael B. Gill and Robert M. Sade, "Paying for Kidneys: The Case against Prohibition," *Kennedy Institute of Ethics Journal* 12, no. 1 (2002).

35. Thomas J Bole III, "The Sale of Organs and Obligations to One's Body: Inferences from the History of Ethics," in *Persons and Their Bodies*, ed. Mark J. Cherry (Boston: Kluwer Academic, 1999).

36. Says Kant, "Man cannot dispose over himself because he is not a thing; he is not his own property; to say that he is would be self-contradictory; for in so far as he is a person he is a Subject in whom the ownership of things can be vested, and if he were his own property, he would be a thing over which he could have ownership. But a person cannot be a property and so cannot be a thing which can be owned, for it is impossible to be a person and a thing, the proprietor and the property. Accordingly, a man is not at his own disposal. He is not entitled to sell a limb, not even one of his teeth." Kant, *Lectures on Ethics*, 165.

37. Harré, "Bodily Obligations."

38. Munzer, "Kant and Property Rights in Body Parts."

39. According to Kant, "The body is part of the self; in its togetherness with the self it constitutes the person." Kant, *Lectures on Ethics*, 166.

40. Munzer, "Kant and Property Rights in Body Parts."

41. Munzer develops a similar response in Munzer, "An Uneasy Case against Property Rights in Body Parts." For another similar treatment, see Gill and Sade, "Paying for Kidneys: The Case against Prohibition."

42. Gerrand, "The Misuse of Kant in the Debate About a Market for Human Body Parts."

43. Cohen, "Public Policy and the Sale of Human Organs." Cohen is actually responding to an argument almost identical in form to the "fallacy of division" argument found in Gill and Sade, "Paying for Kidneys: The Case against Prohibition." Gill and Sade point out that Kant believed that humans possess "dignity" as a consequence of their "humanity." Humanity just is, for Kant, rational nature. Since the sale of kidneys does not harm rational nature, Kant needs an additional argument to show that such sales violate human dignity. While Kantian arguments show what is wrong with selling a whole person or selling any part that destroys the rational nature, they do not succeed in showing why it is wrong to sell parts that don't.

44. Jean-Christophe Merle, "A Kantian Argument for a Duty to Donate One's Own Organs. A Reply to Nicole Gerrand," *Journal of Applied Philosophy* 17, no. 1 (2000).

45. Merle's attempt to save Kant here is highly dubious for several textual reasons. First, Kant never mentions "freedom of choice" as being the reason for prohibiting organ sales. Second, in his only mature discussion of the ethics of organ removal, Kant calls removal of "integral organs" (such as teeth) a "partial self-murder," (*Doctrine of Virtue* 6:423) which implies that dismemberment of non-vital organs is wrong *for the same reason* that suicide is wrong and not for the categorically different reasons that Merle adduces.

46. Alpinar-Şencan, "Reconsidering Kantian Arguments against Organ Selling."

47. James Stacey Taylor, *Stakes and Kidneys: Why Markets in Human Body Parts Are Morally Imperative* (Burlington, VT: Ashgate Pub., 2005), 149–50.

48. Kant, *Lectures on Ethics*, 116.

49. Taylor makes much of Kant's use of the word "particularly," arguing that it suggests Kant thought that in some cases, circumcision would be allowed even if not life-saving. It seems to me that this puts entirely too much weight on Kant's phrasing, in part because this phrase occurs in Kant's precritical lectures, and also because Kant's discussion is clearly intended to address a difficult case having to do with religious conviction, not primarily to discuss the intricacies of allowable self-mutilation. Note that Kant seems to be asking a rhetorical question here; it is not entirely clear that he is endorsing the circumcision.

50. Ruth Chadwick, "The Market for Bodily Parts: Kant and Duties to Oneself," *Journal of Applied Philosophy* 6, no. 2 (1989).

51. According to Kant, it is wrong to "sell or even give away a tooth." *Doctrine of Virtue*, 6:423.

52. Kass, *Life, Liberty, and the Defense of Dignity: The Challenge for Bioethics*, 1st ed., 184.

53. Munzer, "Kant and Property Rights in Body Parts."

54. Cohen, "Selling Bits and Pieces of Humans to Make Babies: The Gift of the Magi Revisited."; Cohen, "Public Policy and the Sale of Human Organs." Stempsey also cites Cohen approvingly on this point. William E Stempsey, "Organ Markets and Human Dignity: On Selling Your Body and Soul," *Christian Bioethics* 6, no. 2 (2000).

55. Morelli, "Commerce in Organs: A Kantian Critique."

56. In other words, they think Kant would prohibit donations not motivated purely by moral duty.

57. Friedrich Heubel and Nicola Biller-Andorno, "The Contribution of Kantian Moral Theory to Contemporary Medical Ethics: A Critical Analysis," *Medicine, Health Care and Philosophy* 8, no. 1 (2005).

58. *Groundwork*, 4:434.

59. Taylor, *Stakes and Kidneys: Why Markets in Human Body Parts Are Morally Imperative*, 154–55.

60. Gerrand, "The Misuse of Kant in the Debate About a Market for Human Body Parts."; Merle, "A Kantian Argument for a Duty to Donate One's Own Organs. A Reply to Nicole Gerrand."; Taylor, *Stakes and Kidneys: Why Markets in Human Body*

Parts Are Morally Imperative; Alpinar-Şencan, "Reconsidering Kantian Arguments against Organ Selling."

61. Gerrand, "The Misuse of Kant in the Debate About a Market for Human Body Parts."

62. *Doctrine of Virtue*, 6:427.

63. Alpinar-Şencan, "Reconsidering Kantian Arguments against Organ Selling."

64. Cècile Fabre, *Whose Body Is It Anyway? Justice and the Integrity of the Person* (Oxford: Clarendon Press, 2009), 140.

65. Powers, "The Integrity of Body: Kantian Moral Constraints on the Physical Self."

66. Merle, "A Kantian Argument for a Duty to Donate One's Own Organs. A Reply to Nicole Gerrand."

67. Merle, "A Kantian Argument for a Duty to Donate One's Own Organs. A Reply to Nicole Gerrand."

68. Two others, already addressed, also make some minimal claims about the governments who would be intervening in the sales. Engelhardt and Gill and Sade both argue some form of the idea that the government should not prohibit sales because Kant failed to establish the existence of moral duties against selling organs. However, because the conclusions in both essays rest on arguments purporting to show Kant's failure to establish the moral duty in question, they seemingly presuppose the idea that Kantian moral duties *could* be enforced, if they could be demonstrated. These authors do not consider whether the government should enforce moral duties in general, only whether the government should enforce primary moral duties grounded in failed moral arguments. See Engelhardt Jr., "The Body for Fun, Beneficence and Profit: A Variation on a Post-Modern Theme"; Gill and Sade, "Paying for Kidneys: The Case against Prohibition"; Engelhardt, "The Injustice of Enforced Equal Access to Transplant Operations: Rethinking Reckless Claims of Fairness."

69. R. S. Taylor, "Self-Ownership and Transplantable Human Organs," *Public Affairs Quarterly* 21, no. 1 (2007).

70. The argument for Kantian self-ownership is developed in Robert S. Taylor, "A Kantian Defense of Self-Ownership," *Journal of Political Philosophy* 12, no. 1 (2004). Taylor applies this concept of self-ownership to markets in organs the later paper, R. S. Taylor, "Self-Ownership and Transplantable Human Organs," *Public Affairs Quarterly* (2007).

71. Dominic J. C. Wilkinson, "Selling Organs and Souls: Should the State Prohibit 'Demeaning' Practices?," *Journal of Bioethical Inquiry* 1, no. 1 (2004).

72. Specifically, Wilkinson points to two passages from Kant's essay, *On the Common Saying: That May Be Correct in Theory but It Is of No Use in Practice*. Both passages decry paternalism.

73. Bole III, "The Sale of Organs and Obligations to One's Body: Inferences from the History of Ethics."

Chapter 4

Kantian Moral Theory and the Problem of Political Legitimacy

Bioethics, I have argued, must address basic questions about what makes government just or legitimate or good if it is to give normative justifications for health laws or policies. In the microcosm of Kantian bioethics literature on organ markets, we have seen how little attention gets paid to such questions in practice.

In this chapter I explore the conceptual problems with basing an account of government on the Kantian account of primary moral duties, which is contained in his moral philosophy. It is perhaps because bioethicists employing Kantian moral principles are steeped in a field that judges laws by whether they enforce moral duties, that Kantian bioethicists have also thought it appropriate to evaluate laws on the basis of Kantian moral principles. But this approach is particularly indefensible from a Kantian perspective. Kant's principles for determining the content of our primary moral duties—the three formulations of the Categorical Imperative—contain within themselves conceptual limitations that prevent their use for directly legitimating laws, policies, or other activities of governments. These conceptual limitations undermine the plausibility of any attempt to justify laws and policies by appealing to Kantian moral duties, such as those described in chapter 3.

Not only do these conceptual limitations preclude the use of the Categorical Imperative in justifying law and policy, they actually pose three substantial challenges to the possibility of explaining how laws can be morally justified *at all*. Any plausible Kantian account of political legitimacy must take these challenges seriously if it is to explain how it is possible to make, interpret, and enforce law without running afoul of the Categorical Imperative.

In this chapter I will focus on the nature of the challenges presented by Kant's moral theory when it is rightly understood. Kant himself understood the problems with applying the Categorical Imperative directly to laws and policies, and I will rely to some extent on his account about why it is not possible to justify laws by appealing directly to Kantian moral duties. The challenges I outline in this chapter will be the benchmark for assessing Kant's own account of legitimacy which I will describe in chapters 5 and 6. I will argue there that Kant's political philosophy largely succeeds in explaining legitimacy in a way that meets the challenges imposed by his moral philosophy.

We will begin with a discussion of the basic problem of political legitimacy, a standard problem in political philosophy and one which requires a normative explanation from any standpoint. Then we will consider several challenges associated with solving the problem of legitimacy, specifically those that can be inferred from Kant's account of moral obligation contained in his discussion of the Categorical Imperative.

THE PROBLEM OF POLITICAL LEGITIMACY

The Basic Problem

The basic problem involved in explaining what makes government just or legitimate or good is that governments routinely act—and claim authority to act—in ways that private persons cannot and do not. Governments make and interpret laws. They incentivize compliance with laws by attaching sanctions to them. And they utilize coercion against those who would resist complying with laws or submitting to penalties for failure to comply.

Governments also seek to exercise a monopoly on the rightful performance of all these actions within a jurisdiction. This attempt to exercise a monopoly is perhaps the most characteristic feature of governments. Some of the features associated with governmental action—making rules, or even using coercion to enforce them—may be performed by other parties. For example, a nightclub owner might set a dress code and ask a bouncer to enforce it. But insofar as these parties operate in a manner consistent with their legal rights, they do not exercise political power, despite acting in ways superficially similar to those characteristic of governments, because they do not attempt to exercise a monopoly on the making, interpreting, and enforcing of law, nor do they challenge the monopoly of the government.[1] (If they openly challenged this monopoly we would probably understand them as revolutionaries, trying to set up a new government.) Thus, although some of the things that governments do can be similar to things that private parties are permitted to do, the governmental effort to impose a monopoly on making, interpreting, and enforcing law effectively distinguishes it from all private parties. We will call this special activity of government the exercise of political power: wielding political power is attempting to exercise a monopoly within a jurisdiction on the making, interpreting, and enforcing of law.[2]

A fundamentally important question to ask about the exercise of political power is whether it is *legitimate*, that is, whether or when it is morally justified. Answering the problem of legitimacy is a major challenge facing any political philosophy because it requires explaining how a government can be morally justified in doing something we don't generally consider persons to have the moral authority to do.[3]

Legitimacy as a Question of Secondary Duties

Laws or policies created by governments are instances of the exercise of political power. Any particular law is an exercise of political power because, generally speaking, it is a part of the government's activity attempting to exercise such a monopoly. When passing a law, the government understands those laws to replace or invalidate any laws that may conflict made by anyone else. By passing a law, the government intends that it, and only it, is entitled to judge whether the law has been broken; and the government attempts to enforce the law through a series of threats or sanctions it expects to be effective.

What morally justifies any such exercise of political power? One common method of assessing the moral justifiability of laws and policies begins by evaluating the primary moral duties that they regulate. As we saw in chapter 3, many authors in the debate about organ markets have used a Kantian moral principle—such as the Formula of Humanity or the idea of human dignity—to show that laws prohibiting the sale of organs are morally justified.

Although Kantian bioethicists frequently assess the legitimacy of laws and policies by scrutinizing the morality of the behaviors these attempt to govern, this approach faces a serious problem, already mentioned several times: it does not actually address the problem of political legitimacy. Authors in the literature often begin by raising the question about the moral justification of the *government's* action (that is, the law the government is making, interpreting, and enforcing), but then, instead of assessing the morality of the *government's* action, they in fact assess only the morality of the behavior that the government seeks to regulate. Even if it is true that organ sales are immoral, the question about political legitimacy is first and foremost a question about the morality of making and enforcing laws governing these behaviors, not about the morality of the behaviors themselves. Legitimacy is, in other words, a question of secondary duties and rights rather than primary ones. As we saw in the last chapter, several authors in this debate (Taylor,[4] Wilkinson,[5] and Bole[6]) have drawn attention to the makers and enforcers of law rather than to their targets. This refocusing is a basic and necessary consequence of understanding the nature of the problem of legitimacy.

It is possible to read the arguments favoring prohibitions in a way in which these authors are not guilty of simply misunderstanding the problem of legitimacy. It could be that authors who take such a simple approach to showing the legitimacy of laws or policies understand their conclusions to rely on an implicit premise, such as "any law prohibiting immoral behavior is morally justified." To put the argument in a form familiar from chapter 1, then:

Major premise [implicit]: [Any law prohibiting immoral behavior is morally justified]

Minor premise: Organ-selling is an immoral behavior (*via Kant's Formula of Humanity or account of human dignity)

Conclusion: A law prohibiting organ-selling is morally justified.

But the major premise here is far too controversial to be left implicit or untreated. It is not widely accepted that any law prohibiting immoral behavior is necessarily legitimate. Even if these authors rely on a more sophisticated major premise about legitimacy than the one I have supplied here, any general claim about what constitutes legitimacy is substantive and controversial enough that it requires explicit attention, especially in an essay that purports to assess the moral justification of some law or policy.

THREE KANTIAN CHALLENGES TO POLITICAL LEGITIMACY

Any attempt to justify a law or policy must assess the exceptional actions of the government that legislates and enforces them, then, not just the morality of the action targeted by the law or policy. But if the question of legitimacy is one about how the exercise of political power is *morally* justified, it might seem that a moral theory such as Kant's can be usefully employed to determine whether prohibitions on organ sales are justified or not.

I will argue, in what follows, that Kantian moral philosophy actually presents three major challenges to any proposed theory of legitimacy. Bioethicists have not understood or recognized these challenges and the limited ability of Kantian moral philosophy to meet these challenges, and this effectively undermines the arguments of all of the commentators on the relationship of Kant to organ markets described in chapter 3.

Enforcing Moral Duty

I have just argued that laws cannot be morally justified simply by showing that they prohibit some immoral action, and that if bioethicists have been using an implicit account of legitimacy, they should address and defend this as an important premise in any argument about the justifiability of law or policy.

Many commentators in the literature on Kant and organ markets suggest that if there is a Kantian moral duty not to sell one's organs under some conditions, then organ sales can be legally prohibited for that reason.[7] It is possible that those making such arguments suspect or perhaps even are committed to the idea that legitimacy is a function of the relationship between the law and the moral duties of citizens in some respect. Perhaps legitimacy depends directly on enforcement of moral duty: law might be justified by the fact that it makes us fulfill our moral duties, or some subset of them (such as the more serious ones). Or perhaps legitimacy depends in some indirect way on moral duty: perhaps a law can be justified if it can be shown that obeying it makes moral agents more likely to fulfill their moral obligations, teaches them the content of their moral duties, or makes it easier for them to fulfill their moral obligations.

Although views of this sort have some defenders, they are particularly problematic from a Kantian perspective. Kant himself provides several arguments for why legitimacy cannot depend directly on enforcement of moral duty. I will briefly discuss these arguments before offering a few thoughts about why it is also unlikely that legitimacy could depend indirectly on moral duty.

Directly Enforcing Moral Duties

The basic reason for thinking that laws cannot be justified on the grounds that they directly enforce our moral duties is that, on Kant's view, it is not possible to force someone to fulfill their moral duties. This impossibility is a consequence of Kant's particular view of morality, outlined in the *Groundwork*, in which two closely related features of morality rule out the possibility that someone could be forced to fulfill their moral duties.

First, persons cannot be forced to fulfill moral duties because it is not possible to fulfill a moral duty unless one acts on the basis of a law one gives to oneself. In chapter 3 I explained Kant's idea that moral duty, if it exists, must be a categorical imperative—meaning that it must bind unconditionally, irrespective of the agent's ends. If moral duty of the kind that is unconditionally binding is possible, it must proceed from practical reason itself. Only an imperative proceeding from reason itself could make our duties unconditionally binding, since its ability to bind would then depend on the strictures of reason, rather than on the contingent ends persons set for themselves.

In his discussion of the third formulation of the Categorical Imperative, the Formula of Autonomy,[8] Kant argues that the fact that the Categorical Imperative proceeds from practical reason means it is a law we give ourselves. It is a law that we give ourselves because it issues from our own use of practical reason. This is the principle of autonomy of the will,[9] the idea that it is possible for moral agents to act on the basis of laws of practical reason, that is, laws they give to themselves.

Acting on the basis of any other law, by contrast, does not fulfill our moral duties. Laws given to us by others are binding on us only insofar as those others attach rewards or sanctions to them. They are not categorical imperatives, because they bind us only insofar as it is our end to obtain the reward or avoid the sanction that is attached to them. Kant groups all such laws together and says their principle is heteronomy of the will.[10] If I act on the basis of such laws, I act as though ruled by another, since the ultimate source of my action is the will of the party offering the sanctions or rewards (in conjunction with my own "self-love," or interest in achieving the reward or avoiding the sanction).[11]

Kant's point is essentially this: to act on moral duty is essentially to act because we can see for ourselves that something is the right thing to do. In such cases, we act as a law unto ourselves. It is our own practical reason that prescribes the act to us, and not the will of another. The incentives offered by others to fulfill laws that they give us cannot make us fulfill our moral duty, because the only way to fulfill our moral duty is to act on the basis of the laws of practical reason, which are laws we give ourselves.

Moral actions cannot be enforced because states have no means by which to cause us to act on laws we give ourselves. The only means that the state possesses to make people act in any way whatsoever depend for their effectiveness on the fact that they introduce some incentive *other than duty* to those subject to the laws. The state may offer negative incentives in the form of sanctions, or positive incentives in the form of rewards. Political power generally utilizes negative incentives but can, in principle, offer either. However, the incentive associated with moral duty is always only *duty itself.* On the Kantian view, duty is its own reward.[12] The person who is motivated primarily by some incentive other than doing the right thing may look externally like the person who acts for duty's sake. Kant gives the example of the shopkeeper who sells goods to a child for a fair price only because he fears the consequences he would face if it were to be discovered that he overcharged children.[13] On Kant's view the shopkeeper acts in conformity with duty, but not from duty, and so not morally. Ultimately, the government can only offer incentives that successfully motivate certain behaviors but thereby guarantee that those behaviors are not actually moral. At best they can make someone do the right thing for the wrong reason.

Second, and closely related, persons cannot be forced to fulfill their moral duties because fulfilling moral duties requires persons to act for certain reasons or ends, and the coercion associated with enforcing laws can only produce actions. The various formulations of the Categorical Imperative make it clear that fulfilling moral duties requires acting for certain ends. For example, the Formula of Universal Law requires acting only on maxims (that is, subjective principles) that can be willed as a universal law. Because a maxim always states an end in acting (for example: "I will lie *in order to obtain something I want*"), the Formula of Universal Law constrains the ends on which persons can act. Similarly, the Formula of Humanity requires treating others as ends, never merely as a means. On Kant's view, this means that our ends in treating others must always be, on some level, compatible with their ends. Kant confirms the idea that ethics requires acting on the basis of specific ends later in the *Doctrine of Virtue*, where he points out that ethics makes commands only for maxims; it is thus a doctrine of ends.[14] But laws cannot have as their object making us act for specific ends: as Kant argues, coercion to adopt ends is impossible because adopting an end is always an exercise of the will and so is always voluntary.[15] The point of coercion is instead to make someone act in a certain way when it is not their end to do so. Consequently, laws can only be justified by reference to the quality of the actions they require, and not by reference to the quality of the reasons for which people do them.

Kant's arguments here paint a picture that I think is basically familiar to us. Consider, for example, a reckless driver who habitually attains speeds exceeding 30 miles per hour above the posted speed limit in residential neighborhoods in the middle of the afternoon. She drives at these speeds for the thrill, despite knowing it is the hour when children typically walk home from school. When she sees a police car in the distance, however, she slows to the posted speed limit until the police car is out of sight. She slows down entirely because she hopes to avoid a speeding ticket.

During the time the driver is within view of the police car she indisputably fulfills her legal duties. But our understanding of her motivation does influence our moral evaluation of her. Regardless of what we would take as sufficient for "doing one's moral duty," it seems unlikely that responding to a fear of a speeding ticket is sufficient for it.

The speeding driver has fulfilled her legal duty by slowing down, even if it is done for the wrong reason. The fact that it is possible for her to completely fulfill her legal duty (even if the fulfillment is only temporary) for the wrong reason is what makes legal duties distinct, in principle, from moral ones. If persons cannot be forced to fulfill their moral duties, then laws (or other manifestations of political power) cannot be justified directly by the fact that they force people to fulfill their moral duties. To claim otherwise would be "self-contradictory,"[16] if we accept the Kantian account of moral obligation.

Indirectly Promoting Moral Duties

Kant's theory of political legitimacy is not directly based on his account of moral duties, as will become apparent in chapter 5. However, one might think it would be possible to offer a Kantian view of legitimacy that depends indirectly on moral duties. Even if coercing obedience to law cannot directly cause someone to act morally, perhaps laws can bring about moral behaviors in more indirect ways. Perhaps, for example, laws can guide us into moral action or teach us the content of moral action, or perhaps laws can make it easier for us to act morally. For example, both Munzer[17] and Kerstein[18] argue, as we have seen, that there may be nothing objectionable with organ sales per se; but that, nevertheless, permitting such sales may encourage certain morally wrong ideas, such as the idea that the poor are for sale, and so are inherently of less dignity than others. On these views, laws can function something like moral teachers: they can serve as a vivid depiction of the inherent dignity and equality of all, even though (as Munzer and Kerstein admit) sales of organs may not inherently compromise the dignity of anyone.

As a justification for the exercise of political power, such indirect approaches are implausible from a Kantian perspective. This is because such indirect approaches depend on the idea that the exercise of political power can be justified by the fact that it is intended to result in some other person or people acting morally (in the examples provided by Munzer and Kerstein above, by maintaining persons' beliefs in their own inherent dignity). But on the Kantian view it is not clear that the morality of others is a meaningful goal at all. For Kant, a moral action is a *free* action, meaning that it is one that is done simply because it is required by practical reason; it is free of any influence from external incentives, or "sensibility." But whether an individual acts freely—and so morally—or whether an individual acts on sensible impulses, in either case it is always the moral agent who is ultimately responsible for her actions. Insofar as she is considered morally responsible at all for her actions, she is their *author*,[19] the first cause of those actions. If it were possible for moral actions to be *caused* by others, or by circumstances they set into motion, then persons would not be capable of the kind of freedom required by Kantian moral theory.

It is for considerations like these that Kant finds two "ends that are also duties" in the *Doctrine of Virtue*: one's own moral perfection, and the happiness of others. Excluded from this short list is the perfection of others. The moral perfection of others cannot be one of our ends at all, says Kant, because individuals can be *morally* responsible only for their own decisions. According to Kant,

> It is a contradiction for me to make another's perfection my end and consider myself under obligation to promote this. For the perfection of another human being, as a person, consists just in this: that he himself is able to set his end in accordance with his own concepts of duty; and it is self-contradictory to require that I do (make it my duty to do) something that only the other himself can do.[20]

This reasoning is just an extension of the reasoning discussed above that moral actions are only those that proceed from a law that a person gives to himself.

Coercion is the most direct way of attempting to influence behavior, but on the Kantian view it is not different in kind from other less-direct attempts to promote "moral" behavior. While either direct coercion or more indirect approaches may influence behavior in some cases, the behaviors produced in such cases cannot be considered "moral" at all: if causal responsibility is attributed to another, then the individual has not been the free cause of her own action, and so has not acted morally by definition.

Justifying Coercion

Suppose, then, that instead of focusing on the morality of the actions subject to laws, we focus instead on the actions of those who write and enforce them, namely, governments. As I have argued, part of what makes the question of legitimacy difficult is the fact that it requires justifying the actions of those who enforce the law. Instead of asking whether the Categorical Imperative can justify behaviors that are *subject to* the coercion inherent in the exercise of political power, then, perhaps we should ask whether the Categorical Imperative can justify the coercive acts themselves. When are coercive acts morally permissible? As we have seen, a few commentators discussing markets in organs have approached the question about the justifiability of prohibitions by asking whether and under what circumstances the Categorical Imperative can sanction coercive interference with organ sales.[21] Taylor, Wilkinson, and Bole all argue that coercing potential organ-sellers is illegitimate because it violates the Categorical Imperative, either by interfering with free actions or by impugning the dignity of sellers. These authors imply that coercion can be justified in some cases, but not in cases where the object is to intervene in self-regarding actions, such as selling organs. But these authors do not take the Categorical Imperative far enough in these arguments, because the Categorical Imperative seems to suggest far more than this: the exact same arguments that they list suggest that coercion cannot be justified *at all* by the Categorical Imperative, even in cases where it is intended to prevent harm to others.

Let us say that coercion is the "use or threat of force." (We will return to the definition of coercion later, when I discuss two substantially different definitions, but for our purposes right now, it will be best to stick with this relatively simple definition). What, exactly, constitutes "force" is not something we need to discuss in much detail in order to generate a problem for Kantian moral philosophy. Force—whatever it is—when exercised intentionally, is intended to stand in contrast to the will of the party being forced. I would only ever use or threaten force if there were reason for thinking that the person I coerce otherwise would not (or at least, might not) comply with the course of action I prefer him to take. Moreover, the use or threat of force only makes sense if the reason he otherwise will not comply is that he does not will to do so. If someone cannot comply with my preferred course of action, either because he physically cannot, because he is not capable of understanding what I want him to do, or for any other reason, then any coercive threats or acts on my part are futile. The use or threat of force only makes sense if the other will not (or likely will not) comply with some preferred behavior because he does not will to do so.

Because coercion is by definition an action intended to counteract the will of another, it is difficult to see how it can be justified by the Categorical Imperative. As we saw, the Formula of Universal Law (the FUL from here on) requires that moral agents "act only in accordance with that maxim through which you can at the same time will that it become a universal law."[22] The test that Kant sets up here requires that moral agents consider whether they could will *everyone* to act on the maxim that they act on. As we saw in chapter 2, the FUL seems to rule out lying, because the liar cannot will that everyone adopt his maxim "I will lie when I wish to obtain something" as a universal law without thereby making his lie ineffective.

In addition to lying, the FUL also seems to prohibit coercion. The FUL requires that I act only on that maxim I can will to serve as a universal law. But it seems that I cannot will coercion *under any circumstances* as a universal law, because—no matter what the circumstances—there is always at least one person I cannot will to be subject to coercion, namely, me. I cannot will myself to be coerced. If someone is only coerced in the case that they would not otherwise will to do that thing, then if I were to will to be coerced it would no longer be coercion.

Allen Wood objects to this line of reasoning, noting that the FUL does not necessarily require that moral agents be able to will every act required by a law in order to be able to will the law as universally binding, because this would make it impossible for us to will a universal law in the case that it prohibited some of our own "immoral inclinations."[23] Wood does not elaborate much on this argument, but we can imagine an example that expresses his concern: suppose that I consider whether I can will truth telling as a universal law, but I remember that on one occasion I did not tell the truth and so was, on that occasion, not able to will truth telling. Moreover, perhaps in that case the incentive was strong enough that I know I would in all likelihood do the exact same thing in the same circumstances again. If the simple fact that I have in the past failed to will some application of a law (or likely will fail to will it in the future) entailed that I could not "will that it become a universal law," then it is unlikely that any maxim could pass the test contained in the FUL.[24]

But the argument above, that coercion cannot be justified by the FUL, does not rely on any kind of claim about whether I always would, as a matter of fact, will to be coerced; instead, the claim is that it is a logical impossibility for me to will to be coerced. Willing to be coerced is, in other words, a contradiction in conception,[25] since being coerced rules out the possibility of willing it.

Christine Korsgaard argues that the Formula of Humanity prohibits coercion even more clearly than does the FUL. Recall that Kant's Formula of Humanity (FH from here on) requires us to treat humanity as an end, never merely as a means. Humanity, for Kant, is rational nature.[26] Rational nature, as the capacity to set and pursue ends, is treated as an end when the bearers of this capacity are not used as a mere means toward ends they have not set for themselves. As Korsgaard points out, Kant gives two tests to determine whether some action necessarily treats others as a mere means: an action necessarily treats another as a mere means if he "cannot possibly assent to it" and if he "cannot contain the end of this action in himself."[27] As Korsgaard argues, coercion obviously fails both tests: by definition a coercive action is one which the coerced party "cannot possibly assent" to, and is one in which the coerced party "cannot contain the end of the action in himself." Because coercion (along with deception) fails the test, Korsgaard argues that coercion and deception are "the most fundamental forms of wrongdoing to others—the roots of all evil." She concludes that Kant's Categorical Imperative, at least in the FH version,[28] cannot permit any deception or coercion at all. This conclusion should not be entirely surprising. In his essay, "On the Supposed Right to Lie from Philanthropy," Kant argues that deception is immoral even if it is necessary to misdirect a "murderer at the door."[29] The clear implication is that actions that are themselves wrongful do not become justified in any cases at all, not even when they respond to someone else's wrongdoing.

Despite these problems, I do not think the argument given so far conclusively shows that intentional coercion—of the kind present in the enforcement of law—cannot pass the tests required by the Categorical Imperative. In chapter 6 I will offer an argument meant to show that at least some instances of coercive enforcement of law can pass the tests in the FUL and the FH. My argument here is intended only to show that there is no easy or straightforward way to justify coercion, and thus the exercise of political power, based on Kantian moral principles taken at face value. While justifying coercion may not be the first priority of a moral theory—most private agents in basically just societies rarely find themselves in circumstances requiring the exercise of coercion—it does seem to be an important, and likely foundational, element of any plausible political theory. Because the *Groundwork* gives no clear account about when coercion is justified, Kant needs an additional substantial explanation about this if there is to be a Kantian solution to the problem of political legitimacy.

Reconciling Political Power with Moral Equality

There is still another challenge for any Kantian attempt to morally justify the exercise of political power. This challenge arises because of the government's claim to a monopoly in making, interpreting, and enforcing law, which is not easily reconciled with the Kantian commitment to fundamental moral equality.

Assume for the moment that, despite the difficulties just discussed, there is some Kantian solution to the problems that his moral principles seem to present for justifying coercion, and coercion can be morally justified by Kantian moral principles in at least some cases. Perhaps, for example, there is some way of arguing that Kantian moral principles can justify coercion when it is exercised to stop armed assault. Preventing armed assault must rank as among the least controversial uses of coercion, and we might expect that if Kant's moral principles can justify any uses of coercion, they could justify it in this case.

Even if that were true, however, Kantian moral philosophy presents still another challenge for the claim that such coercion could be morally legitimate if exercised by the government. This is because, even in what are seemingly the least controversial cases, governments act coercively in the context of a supposed right to exercise political power. By claiming political power, as I argued earlier, they are not merely claiming a right to use coercion in circumstances where it would be justified for anyone to use. Instead, they claim the right to hold a *monopoly* on the making, interpretation, and enforcement of laws. When government agents use coercion to protect themselves or others from assailants, they do so as an extension of their supposedly exclusive right to define what counts as assault, to judge whether particular cases meet that definition, and to enforce their determinations about this. By claiming such a monopoly on the making, interpreting, and enforcing of the law, the government claims a right to treat citizens in ways that they cannot reciprocate. This seems to make them unequal to one another.

Kant does not explicitly discuss equality in the *Groundwork*, but the idea of moral equality is fundamental to Kant's moral theory, both in the *Groundwork* and elsewhere. For example, the idea that persons are subject to laws they could will as *universal* contains the idea of equality: any true law of morality is one that could hold equally for all rational beings. To will something for other rational beings, but not for oneself, is to make an exception of oneself;[30] it is to treat oneself as morally unequal. Similarly, by prohibiting treatment of others as mere means, the Formula of Humanity also assumes that persons are fundamentally morally equal, because they are equally entitled to pursue their own ends and not be made subject to the ends of others. Their moral value can be expressed as a "dignity beyond price," a value that accrues equally to persons because they possess rational nature.

The exceptional powers and rights claimed by the government cannot be easily reconciled with this fundamental moral equality. The government has the power to make laws that bind me, to interpret those laws when there is a dispute about them, and to enforce those laws if I do not obey them. In contrast, I have no such authority to do these things to the government. What justifies this inequality? In a democratic society, it might seem plausible to point out that the government was democratically chosen, so I had an equal chance to vote on the people occupying these positions. But this response only serves to raise further questions. In a democratic political system, the legislators (and so the laws, in some respect) are chosen by vote. But at the end of the day, such votes always involve one group (usually, the majority) selecting the legislators, and so indirectly making the rules to which everyone is subject. Even if we conceive of legislators as the instruments of the majority, there is still an equality problem: why should I be subject to the determinations of other citizens, just because they are in the majority?

Of course, if I had agreed to be bound by the will of the majority, it might preserve my equality. Suppose I enter into an agreement with you that we shall play a game, where the winner gets to choose where we eat for dinner. If I lose the game and you get to choose where we eat, the decision about where we eat is made unequally, but it poses no challenge to our *moral* equality. I agreed to be bound by such a rule and treating me as a moral equal seems to require taking my consent (or lack thereof) as determinative in most matters concerning me. However, in the case of laws I never agreed to be bound by the will of the majority or by any of the major rules or institutions exercising political power in my society. Most of these were established long before I was born. Any Kantian response to the legitimacy problem must reconcile this apparent inequality with a more fundamental commitment to moral equality between all persons.

The challenge from equality is the final nail in the coffin of attempts to legitimate laws or policies by simple implementation of moral principles, such as the various formulations of the Categorical Imperative. Even if it were possible to meet the first two challenges, we would still be a long way from explaining the moral justification of law. Because laws are written, interpreted, and enforced within the context of the government's overall attempt to exercise political power, we need a further account to explain how such moral powers are possible, given Kantian commitments to moral equality. What we need, in other words, is an account of legitimacy, not just morally justified coercion.

From Moral to Political Principles

Kant's moral philosophy, then, poses several challenges to any possible Kantian solution to the problem of political legitimacy. A Kantian solution to the problem of legitimacy must, in the first place, justify law without making the justification dependent on enforcing the fulfillment of moral duties, or even indirectly promoting them. It must, further, explain how coercion is morally possible, given the apparent condemnation of all coercive acts by the various formulations of the Categorical Imperative. And any Kantian solution to the problem of legitimacy must, ultimately, achieve this explanation without abandoning fundamental moral equality between those who wield political power and those who are subject to it. Taken together, these limitations present a stiff challenge to those would use the principles in the familiar *Groundwork* to reach conclusions about the legitimacy of governmental activities. As we have seen in our survey of the bioethics literature on Kant and organ markets, most efforts to justify laws or policies based on Kant's moral principles fail to take seriously one or more of these limitations, already apparent from a careful reading of the *Groundwork*.

Kant himself developed an account of political legitimacy that takes seriously the limitations implicit in the *Groundwork*. This account of legitimacy is presented in his political philosophy, not his moral philosophy, and is found most definitively in the *Doctrine of Right*, which composes the first half of his most mature work on practical philosophy, the *Metaphysics of Morals*. There Kant develops political principles to justify the exercise of political power. These political principles form Kant's theory of justice or the "doctrine of right." Kant argues that the domain of justice or "right" should be considered distinct in principle from the domain of moral obligation, alternatively referred to as the "doctrine of virtue" and "ethics." In chapters 5 and 6 I will trace Kant's answer to the legitimacy problem and argue that it largely succeeds in solving that problem without running afoul of the limitations.

It might seem natural to think that these political principles must, despite their distinction from moral obligation, be an extension of Kant's moral principles as found in the *Groundwork*. As I have suggested, solving the legitimacy problem requires showing that the exercise of political power is *morally* justified, and this would seem to require some explanation—perhaps something more sophisticated than that usually employed by contemporary commentators—of how coercion can be justified with reference to the Categorical Imperative. I have argued that the Categorical Imperative actually poses significant difficulties for any justification of coercion, but surely this is nevertheless the bar that Kant must meet in order to solve the problem of legitimacy.

As we will see, however, Kant does not clearly depend on the Categorical Imperative in any of its forms in his account of legitimacy. Although Kant has much to say about the relationship between morality and justice, Kant does not clearly derive his principles of justice from the Categorical Imperative, or even discuss how his principles of justice are related to the Categorical Imperative. This has caused problems for Kantian moral theorists because it means that the relationship between Kant's moral and political theory is ambiguous.[31]

This ambiguity need not pose a problem for the present purposes, however. The purpose in this chapter has been to show why it is that Kantian moral philosophy is not readily or directly applicable in the justification of laws or policies. His moral philosophy is intended to explain the nature of moral duty and its relationship to practical reason, not to deal specifically with the special problems raised by the exercise of political power. Kant himself saw this and developed a political philosophy in answer to the problem of political legitimacy. The precise nature of the relationship between his moral and political philosophy is an important question, but beyond the scope of our discussion. A treatment paying special attention to the problem of political legitimacy is necessitated by his moral theory, and that is something that Kant, but not his contemporary interpreters, appreciated. In what follows I will assess Kant's account of legitimacy on its own merits, although we will return to the question about how coercion can be reconciled with the Categorical Imperative in chapter 6.

NOTES

1. On this definition, the nightclub owner and bouncer would exercise political power if they attempted to exercise a monopoly on these elements within the nightclub. If the attempt to exercise the monopoly conflicted with the government's laws or policies, the government would presumably treat this as criminal activity. We often

presume that criminal activity is less morally justified than the attempt to prevent it; but of course, in this case, without any further details about the government's laws, or the alternative proposed by the nightclub owner, it is impossible to reach any conclusion on whose attempt at enforcing a monopoly on making, interpreting, and enforcing law is morally justified (if either). The nightclub would simply pose a threat to the government's monopoly, and so would in that sense be an exercise of political power.

2. This discussion closely follows the account of political power in Allen Buchanan, "Political Legitimacy and Democracy," *Ethics* 112, no. 4 (2002).

3. For a discussion of this, see Michael Huemer, *The Problem of Political Authority: An Examination of the Right to Coerce and the Duty to Obey* (New York: Palgrave Macmillan, 2013), Ch. 1.

4. Robert S. Taylor, "Self-Ownership and Transplantable Human Organs," *Public Affairs Quarterly* 21, no. 1 (2007).

5. Dominic J. C. Wilkinson, "Selling Organs and Souls: Should the State Prohibit 'Demeaning' Practices?," *Journal of Bioethical Inquiry* 1, no. 1 (2004).

6. Thomas J Bole III, "The Sale of Organs and Obligations to One's Body: Inferences from the History of Ethics," in *Persons and Their Bodies*, ed. Mark J. Cherry (Boston: Kluwer Academic, 1999).

7. For example, Ruth Chadwick, "The Market for Bodily Parts: Kant and Duties to Oneself," *Journal of Applied Philosophy* 6, no. 2 (1989); Leon R Kass, "Organs for Sale? Propriety, Property, and the Price of Progress," *The Public Interest*, no. 107 (1993); Ronald M Green, "What Does It Mean to Use Someone as 'a Means Only': Rereading Kant," *Kennedy Institute of Ethics Journal* 11, no. 3 (2001); Cynthia B Cohen, "Public Policy and the Sale of Human Organs," *Kennedy Institute of Ethics Journal* 12, no. 1 (2002); Leon Kass, *Life, Liberty, and the Defense of Dignity: The Challenge for Bioethics*, 1st ed. (San Francisco: Encounter Books, 2002); Mario Morelli, "Commerce in Organs: A Kantian Critique," *Journal of Social Philosophy* 30, no. 2 (2004); Samuel Kerstein, "Autonomy, Moral Constraints, and Markets in Kidneys," *Journal of Medicine and Philosophy* 34, no. 6 (2009); Samuel Kerstein, "Kantian Condemnation of Commerce in Organs," *Kennedy Institute of Ethics Journal* 19, no. 2 (2009); Susan M. Shell, "Kant's Concept of Human Dignity," in *Human Dignity and Bioethics*, ed. Edmund D. Pellegrino et al. (Notre Dame, Ind.: University of Notre Dame Press, 2009).

8. Formula of Autonomy: "The idea of the will of every rational being as a will giving universal law." *Groundwork*, 4:431.

9. *Groundwork*, 4:433.

10. *Groundwork*, 4:433.

11. On Kant's view it is possible, I take it, to obey someone else and act morally. For example, in chapter 6 I will discuss how the government can come to have moral authority as an exercise of a general and united will. However, the *ultimate* reason for obeying the other cannot be the incentive that that person has attached to obedience. It is only possible for me to fulfill a moral duty by obeying someone else if I obey the other on the basis of a law I have given myself, that is, if I act autonomously rather than heteronomously. In this case, it is ultimately I myself who gives the law, even if the duty may be mediated by an external lawgiver. As Kant puts it,

in such cases I am the "supreme lawgiver" (*Groundwork*, 4:432). Moreover, in such cases the incentive to act is duty itself, and not the incentive offered by the lawgiver. So it would be a misnomer to say that the person who obeys, in this situation, has been forced to act morally. They would have acted morally even without the incentive.

12. *Doctrine of Virtue*, 6:396.
13. *Groundwork*, 4:397.
14. *Doctrine of Virtue*, 6:410
15. *Doctrine of Virtue*, 6:381
16. *Doctrine of Virtue*, 6:381
17. Stephen R Munzer, "An Uneasy Case against Property Rights in Body Parts," *Social Philosophy and Policy* 11, no. 2 (1994).
18. Kerstein, "Autonomy, Moral Constraints, and Markets in Kidneys"; Kerstein, "Kantian Condemnation of Commerce in Organs."
19. Immanuel Kant, "The Doctrine of Right," in *The Metaphysics of Morals*, ed. and trans. Mary J. Gregor (New York: Cambridge University Press, 1996), 6:223. Further references to the *Doctrine of Right* are indicated by page numbers only and refer to this edition. All references to Kant's works use the Prussian Academy pagination.
20. *Doctrine of Virtue*, 6:386
21. Bole III, "The Sale of Organs and Obligations to One's Body: Inferences from the History of Ethics."; Wilkinson, "Selling Organs and Souls: Should the State Prohibit 'Demeaning' Practices?"; Taylor, "Self-Ownership and Transplantable Human Organs."
22. *Groundwork*, 4:421.
23. Allen Wood, "Right and Ethics: Arthur Ripstein's Force and Freedom," in *Freedom and Force: Essays on Kant's Legal Philosophy*, ed. Sari Kisilevsky and Martin Jay Stone (Portland, OR: Hart Publishing, 2017), 164.
24. Kant himself addresses this objection in his discussion of the golden rule (*Groundwork*, 4:430). He points out there that a judge could not sentence a criminal if it were the case that the FUL prohibited treating others in ways that we would not want to be treated. Kant suggests in the example that it is permissible for the judge to sentence the criminal because the criminal *could* contain the end of punishment in himself, even though he doesn't *actually* want to be punished. Although Kant suggests it is possible for the criminal to consent to punishment, he does not explain *how* it is possible to will to be subject to coercion here. We will return to this question in chapter 6.
25. Kant discusses two kinds of contradictions that can emerge when we attempt to universalize our maxims. Contradictions in conception occur when actions are "so constituted that their maxim cannot even be thought without contradiction as a universal law of nature," while contradictions in the will occur when it is "impossible to will that [an action's] maxim be raised to the universality of a law of nature because such a will would contradict itself." *Groundwork*, 4:424.
26. *Groundwork*, 4:437
27. *Groundwork*, 4:429–30

28. Korsgaard, contra Kant, holds that the FUL and FH are not equivalent. Moreover, she argues that the FUL could allow lying in some circumstances—specifically, those circumstances in which the lie is something that one could will in all similar situations and the recipient of the lie does not know that one is in such circumstances (which is necessary for preventing the lie from being ineffective if universally willed). See Christine Korsgaard, "The Right to Lie: Kant on Dealing with Evil," *Philosophy and Public Affairs* 15, no. 4 (1986).

29. Immanuel Kant, "On a Supposed Right to Lie from Philanthropy," in *Practical Philosophy*, ed. and trans. Mary J. Gregor, The Cambridge Edition of the Works of Immanuel Kant (New York: Cambridge University Press, 1996).

30. *Groundwork,* 4:424

31. Some commentators argue that Kant's political philosophy can be derived from his moral philosophy. See Onora O'Neill, "Kant and the Social Contract Tradition," in *Kant Actuel: Hommage À Pierre Laberge*, ed. François Duchesneau, Claude Piché, and Guy Lafrance (Montréal: Bellarmin, 2000); Gerhard Seel, "How Does Kant Justify the Universal Objective Validity of the Law of Right?," *International Journal of Philosophical Studies* 17, no. 1 (2009); Louis Philippe Hodgson, "Kant on the Right to Freedom: A Defense," *Ethics* 120, no. 4 (2010); Japa Pallikkathayil, "Deriving Morality from Politics: Rethinking the Formula of Humanity," *Ethics* 121, no. 1 (2010). Others have argued that Kant's political philosophy is suggested by his moral philosophy, but that it also stands independently. See Thomas W. Pogge, "Is Kant's Rechtslehre Comprehensive?," *The Southern Journal of Philosophy* 36, no. S1 (1998); Arthur Ripstein, *Force and Freedom: Kant's Legal and Political Philosophy* (Cambridge, Mass.: Harvard University Press, 2009), Appendix. Still others have argued that the two are probably incompatible. See Marcus Willaschek, "Why the Doctrine of Right Does Not Belong in the Metaphysics of Morals," *Annual Review of Law and Ethics* 5 (1997); Allen W. Wood, "The Final Form of Kant's Practical Philosophy," *Southern Journal of Philosophy* 36 (1997).

Chapter 5

Rights as the Basis for Political Legitimacy

SOLVING THE PROBLEM OF LEGITIMACY

In the *Groundwork*, as we have now seen, Kant is concerned with the concept of moral duty. In his political philosophy, however, Kant begins with what he calls the "concept of right." Beginning with right instead of duty offers several advantages to Kant, some of which I will outline here. My strategy will be to follow Kant's analysis of the concept of right and to show how he uses this to develop the most basic principle for justifying the exercise of political power, the Universal Principle of Right. This principle undergirds Kant's political philosophy, but I will focus in this chapter on explaining how it follows from the concept of right and how it can justify basic cases of coercion. This account will not be a full explanation of political legitimacy, however, because justifying the exercise of political power requires more than simply justifying coercion. An account of political legitimacy must also justify exercising a monopoly on making, interpreting, and enforcing law. The remainder of Kant's justification of political power, including the exercise of a monopoly on these further elements, will be the subject of chapter 6. The full account of political legitimacy, I will argue, solves the basic problem of legitimacy while also meeting all three of the stiff challenges posed by Kant's moral philosophy.

The task in this chapter and the next is not primarily a defense of Kant's political philosophy.[1] I will offer a few comments comparing Kant's theory to contemporary theories, but the main agenda for these chapters is to develop the account of political legitimacy that we said is necessitated by, but not provided in, Kant's moral philosophy, and to show how it is compatible with his moral philosophy. This account of political legitimacy will then be the basis

RIGHT AND JUSTIFIED ACTION

Method: Intuition or Analysis?

In contemporary moral and political philosophy, philosophers will sometimes begin with intuitions and considered judgments about what seems "just" in particular cases, and then move on from there to select various principles that can explain those intuitions. Through a process of reflective equilibrium, principles can thus be slowly developed to bring consistency between considered judgments about cases and the principles that constitute an overall political framework.

Kant's method is different. Although he does at times appeal to the intuitions of his audience, his method begins by analyzing a familiar concept, and then reasoning to the conditions for the possibility of such a concept—a method referred to as a "transcendental argument."[2] This method may be familiar to readers of the *Groundwork*, for example, where Kant begins with the familiar concepts of a "good will" and "moral duty,"[3] and then reasons from there to the existence and content of a supreme principle of morality. In the *Doctrine of Right*, instead of beginning with moral duty Kant begins with the concept of right (*Recht*), which is the concept at the root of individual rights (as well as some other things, less familiar to us perhaps[4]), and reasons from there to basic principles explaining government legitimacy and authority.

Beyond fitting well with his overall critical method, by beginning with a concept that is familiar from our everyday moral discourse, Kant's approach is promising because it does not begin with contested intuitions. This can be valuable for political philosophy, I think, in part because "intuitions" about what makes governments just or legitimate or good are extremely divergent. Instead, Kant begins with a familiar concept and then asks about the implications of that concept correctly understood. We shall begin our treatment at Kant's starting point, with his analysis of right.

The Concept of Right

On Kant's analysis, the concept of right has three distinctive features which progressively sharpen our picture of it.

Relationships

At its base, the concept of right is about the relationship between persons. Says Kant, "the moral concept of right . . . has to do, first, only with the external and indeed practical relation of one person to another insofar as their actions, as deeds, can have (direct or indirect) influence on each other."[5] The relational aspect of right follows from the fact that a rights-claim is fundamentally moral in nature: an entity against whom we can have a right must, necessarily, be an entity capable of acting morally. We cannot have rights against cars, mountains, the weather, infants, or animals, insofar as these are not capable of responding to any moral demands we might make of them. The relational aspect of right illustrates something not always apparent in contemporary discussions about distributive justice, which often focus on the specific goods to which people are entitled. The tenor of these discussions sometimes suggests that the most important questions about rights are questions about the relationship between persons and things—for example, the goods persons need, or the goods that they would want, whatever else they want (such as wealth, income, or health care). But because the concept of right is fundamentally about a relationship between persons, any claim that persons have a right to some good necessarily relies—sometimes implicitly or even unconsciously—on the existence of a person or party who is obligated to provide that good. Without a moral agent or party that is the recipient of the rights claim, a rights claim would be meaningless.

Choice

More specifically, the concept of right is about only one aspect of the relationship between persons: the way in which their choices impact one another. According to Kant, "choice" refers to the exercise of (or a decision against the exercise of) an existing capacity to bring about an end. In this way a choice is different from a wish: we wish for something when we do not have the capacity to bring it about.[6] We make a choice when we take up means toward ends; lacking the means to move toward some end, we may wish for the end, but we cannot make a choice about it. We cannot even choose not to pursue it, since we make no meaningful choice when we lack the means to pursue it.

The concept of right is concerned with choices, rather than wishes, because choices bring us into relationship with one another in a way that needs or wishes do not. By using means to achieve my ends, I affect the means available to you, and so the choices that you have. Because wishes and needs need not result in action, they may not affect others at all. They only affect our relationship with others insofar as we take up means to pursue them. So the concept of right has to do with the relationship between the choice of one and the choice of another—specifically, it is concerned with whether and to what extent our use of means impacts or influences the means available to others.

This does not mean that the content of rights could not, in some cases, be defined relative to needs or wishes. If that were true, then persons could not have welfare rights based on their needs, for example, a view that Kant rejects elsewhere.[7] However, it does mean that needs or wishes are not essential to the concept of right. A right can always be described purely in terms of how the choices of one may affect the choices of another, without any reference to the needs or wishes of either party. On Kant's analysis, this is the more basic and general use of the concept of right.

Freedom

However, the concept of right is not mere description of the ways in which one person's choices might impact another's. Instead, right is the idea that it is possible for each person's choices to be free of the choices of others, under universal law.[8]

That right is fundamentally concerned with freedom is familiar. Sometimes rights are about active freedoms, such as a freedom to move or associate, or a freedom to alter another's duties. Sometimes rights are about passive freedoms, such as being free from interference or free from another's authority.[9] But what does it mean to be free? "Free" can mean many different things, depending on the context. When we talk about the freedom associated with rights, we mean that we have discretion over something. This is what makes rights fundamentally different from duties: to have a duty is to lack discretion over something, or to be bound with respect to it. For example, to have a right to speak freely is to have discretion about whether to speak and what to say. To have a duty not to speak is to lack this discretion.

This is so even when we think of a right to some specific good, such as a right to a piece of property, or a right to adequate nutrition or housing. Although speaking about a "right" to such things might seem to suggest that we have some special relationship to the things themselves, the right we have to these things is better understood as a right to discretion in how we use or dispose of such things, free from interference by others. I have a right to a piece of property if that property is used at my discretion, rather than at the discretion of someone else. I have a right to adequate nutrition or housing if I have discretion over whether I receive those benefits, such that if I decide I want them, others are bound to give them to me. In each case choice is free in the sense that no one else can impede my choice or tell me whether or how I must act within the realm of my discretion.

According to Kant, the kind of freedom with which right is concerned is what we might call *external* freedom. External freedom is markedly different from the metaphysical concept of "free choice" familiar from Kant's moral philosophy (and important as a background concept in Kant's political philosophy as well[10]). As we saw in chapter 4, Kant argues in the *Groundwork* that persons are capable of acting on the basis of pure practical reason—basically, acting on the moral law—rather than on the basis of various interests that would otherwise motivate us. He describes this as acting on *reason,* rather than *inclination.*[11] However, external freedom (or, as Kant puts it, "freedom in the external use of choice"[12]) means, essentially, being free of others' interfering choices.[13] To say that a choice is externally "free" is to say nothing about the reasons for which it is performed, then, but only to say that others did not interfere with it.

External freedom is not possible in any absolute sense in our world, because the earth is physically bounded and other people exist on it. My choices are never entirely externally free so long as people have altered the physical world in which I make those choices. I can, however, be free of specific kinds of choices by others. A law defining the specific ways in which I am free of others' choices can create for me, essentially, a normative domain in which I am free. For example, a law might endow me with a right to choose whether and when others touch me (with some exceptions, perhaps, such as when I have broken a law or am unconscious and in need of emergency treatment). The choices I subsequently make about who may touch my body are not entirely externally or empirically free, in the sense of "completely unaffected by the actions of others": my choices about who may touch me may still be affected by their choices, for example, about what to offer me in return (I might consent to be touched, for example, by a surgeon who promises to heal me); or their choices to make my life more difficult in a number of ways, if I do not consent (an employer might threaten to replace me if I will not consent to periodic virus or drug tests). Even so, a law prohibiting touching my body without my consent preserves a domain for me in which I am free of specific kinds of choices made by others. Such a law effectively makes me free in a specific sense from the influence of their choices, even if I am still affected by their choices in other ways. Although laws cannot insulate me entirely from the choices of others—we cannot be *completely* insulated from the choices of others so long as we share time and space with them—they can carve out a realm in which I may make choices that are guaranteed to be insulated from specific kinds of choices by others. My right to refuse the touch of others is a vivid example of just how meaningful and significant such a limited domain of freedom can be.

Consequently, in a bounded world with other people in it, the possibility of any freedom of choice depends on a law that circumscribes this freedom. Any such law must be, additionally, universal, in the sense that it carves out the same kind of domain of freedom for everyone else, as well. This follows from the basically moral nature of rights: as moral powers, moral agents must possess them equally. Insofar as the concept of right carves out a domain of freedom for one person, then, the moral nature of the concept requires that it must also carve out a domain of freedom for everyone, circumscribed by the same law.

Because right is fundamentally about defining a domain of external freedom where our choices are free of influence from others, it is silent about the reasons for which we act or the ends we have when we act. Because having a right means being free (in some defined sense) of influence by the choices of others, the concept of right is fundamentally about circumscribing a domain in which people may act according to their *own* ends rather than the ends of others. Consequently, Kant says that right is about the *form* of the relation between choices—that is, the way in which an action affects another's external freedom—and not the *matter* of choice, that is, the ends for which a choice is made.[14]

This is not to say that the ends of an action could not be made relevant to the rightfulness of a choice. For example, establishing that a crime has been committed usually requires establishing a *mens rea* ("guilty mind"), meaning that the defendant intended to commit the crime. In this sense committing the crime was the criminal's "end" (whatever the ultimate end may have been). Instead, the argument is that ends are not a feature of the concept of right itself, even if in some cases we make rights relative to specific ends. And this is familiar to us: property rights, rights to free speech, and many other rights all function to protect persons in activities whose ends are chosen only by themselves. The existence of the right does not depend on the ends of the person who owns the property or who participates in political speech, nor does it depend on the ends of those who might wish to interfere with these rights. If it did, it would no longer be meaningful to talk about having a "right" to these things at all.

The concept of right, then, refers ultimately to a relationship between persons, where each enjoys a domain of choices, free from influence by the choices of others, as circumscribed under a set of universal laws.

Rights in Context

Although it is outside the scope of this discussion to argue that Kant's account of rights is correct, it is worth briefly putting Kant's theory of rights in the context of contemporary rights theory. Following Wenar,[15] we can compare Kant's theory of rights to other theories of rights by considering first the form of Kantian rights and then their function.

First, with respect to the form of rights, on Kant's account a "right" signifies a relationship between persons, in which one party is free to make some choice, independent of the choices of the other (or others). This account has much in common with Hohfeld's analysis of rights,[16] widely accepted in contemporary rights discourse.[17] In Hohfeld's account, rights denote one of four kinds of relations between the right-holder and other persons. For each of the Hohfeldian incidents, the right-holder is free to make a choice independent of the choices of others. The kind of choice that the right-holder possesses falls into one of four categories. All four categories can be understood as compatible with the Kantian account of rights, and Kant discusses examples of each over the course of his political writings.[18]

Kant has less to say about the function of rights. Contemporary discussion is divided about whether the function of rights is to allow the right-holder to alter the duties of others (the will theory of rights) or whether the function of rights is to protect important interests (the interest theory of rights). Although Kant is sometimes read as espousing the will theory of rights,[19] his analysis of rights does not strictly tell us what the function or purpose of rights is; instead, it merely describes the relationship entailed by rights.

This is not to say that Kant's theory, taken as a whole, will be consistent with both the will and interest theories of rights. It probably isn't compatible with either theory, all things considered. This basic inconsistency stems from the fact that both theories assume that rights have a single moral purpose, that is, they exist to achieve some good external to themselves (either to make possible relations of authority or to protect important interests). Instead, in the Kantian analysis, rights are simply a feature of our moral lives: they express a specific moral relationship between persons, and they exist as a function of the fact that we are equally free. Importantly, however, they do not exist because of the value or importance of protecting our freedom. Instead, rights exist because others, as our moral equals, lack the authority to bind us in ways that we cannot bind them.[20]

Rights and Duties of Right

The concept of right explains what it means for one person to *have a right* against another (or others in general): to have such a right is to have some choice that is free of the other's choices in some way, circumscribed under universal law. But it also explains what it means for a condition among persons to be characterized by right, as in a *rightful condition*: such a condition is one in which universal laws make the free choice of each compatible with the external freedom of all. Thirdly, it can explain what it means for an individual action to be a *rightful action*. As Kant puts it, "Any action is right if it can coexist with everyone's freedom in accordance with a universal law."[21] From this definition of rightful actions, a definition of non-rightful ones follows: an action will be wrong if it *cannot* coexist with everyone's freedom, or as Kant puts it, if it acts as a "hindrance" or "resistance" to freedom in accordance with a universal law.[22]

The primary political principle, or duty, of Kant's *Doctrine of Right* is developed from this understanding of a wrong action. If a wrong action is any action that cannot coexist with the freedom of others under universal law, then the primary political duty is the duty not to commit such wrong actions. The Universal Principle of Right, accordingly, commands: "So act externally that the free use of your choice can coexist with the freedom of everyone in accordance with a universal law."

RIGHTFUL AND WRONGFUL COERCION

Coercion as a Hindrance to Freedom

Coercion, on the Kantian account, is any "hindrance to freedom."[23] This definition bears a crucial similarity to the one discussed in chapter 4, the idea of the "use or threat of force." A use or threat of force, as discussed earlier, always is intended to frustrate or hinder another person's freedom. There would be no reason to force someone to do something that you expected them to do or that they had already consented to do. Force is offered precisely because someone may not act freely in the desired way.

However, Kant's definition of coercion departs from common understandings of coercion in at least three ways. We shall return to examine these differences later in the chapter. But for now, let us note the distinctive features of Kant's view. First, if a coercive act is any hindrance to freedom, then an action need not be effective in deterring someone, nor likely to deter someone, to count as coercion. To some authors, the expectation of success determines whether an action is coercive. For example, brandishing an AK-47 to steal someone's wallet seems coercive, but brandishing a water pistol for the same purpose does not. On Kant's definition, even the water pistol could count as coercive, although the hindrance to keeping one's wallet is obviously much less significant in the latter case than it is the former.

Similarly, if coercion is *any* hindrance to freedom, then coercion need not be strictly intended to coerce *at all*. Many of the actions we perform may force others to behave in a certain way, or at least make it more likely that they will, without being intended to have that effect. I may build a fence around my backyard to keep the dogs or the kids inside, or I may build it to achieve a "white picket fence" look, without ever considering the fact that it also constrains those who would enter my property without my permission. Because coercion is a hindrance to *freedom,* actions are coercive even if they constrain others from making choices they were unlikely to make or did not want to make anyway. I can constrain your freedom by cutting off options, even if those are options you would not have taken and even if I do not think it likely that you would take them. My fence functions as a constraint on the Queen of England, even though there is no reason for thinking it likely that she will try to trespass on my property.

Finally, because coercion is *any* hindrance to freedom in accordance with universal law, coercion is not a moralized term. In this way it is different from standard uses in the bioethics literature, where it is sometimes used to explain a fundamental wrong-making feature of certain kinds of actions.[24] But on Kant's account, coercion is *any* hindrance to freedom, and so does not carry with it any connotation of wrongdoing.

Justifying Coercion

The justifiability of coercion, on Kant's account, is ultimately determined by whether the coercive action is right or wrong. It is determined in exactly the same way that the justifiability of every other kind of action is: not by whether it hinders freedom, but by whether the freedom it hinders is a freedom *in accordance with a universal law*. Any hindrance to such freedom is wrong; this follows, necessarily, from the fact that *any action* that cannot coexist with everyone's freedom in accordance with a universal law is wrong.

Coercion can also be rightful, on the same argument. While an action that hinders freedom under universal law is wrong, an action that counteracts such an action—as Kant puts it, a "hindering of a hindrance to freedom"[25]—is consistent with freedom under universal law, and so is right. This follows from the definition of a right action given earlier: *any* action is right if it can coexist with the freedom of everyone in accordance with universal law. If a coercive act could coexist with the freedom of everyone under universal law but was nevertheless *wrong,* this would contradict the previously given definition for right action.

On Kant's account, then, coercive acts are justified by the fact that they can be understood as merely rightful, as expressions of freedom consistent with the freedom of others under universal law.

This justification has several important consequences for our understanding of rightful coercion. First, the ends of the coercer do not affect the justifiability of a coercive act. I argued previously that ends don't matter for determining whether an act is coercive; all that matters is whether the action is a hindrance to freedom. Similarly, ends don't make a difference to the justifiability of a coercive act: if my act is consistent with the freedom of everyone under universal law, then it is justifiable even if I did it for the wrong reasons. I might erect a white fence because I like it, or I might do it simply because I know it will annoy you; what matters is whether my action can coexist with the freedom of everyone under universal law, and not whether my ends are morally worthy or not.

Second, the effect of my coercive action on your interests also does not matter for determining whether the coercion is justified. I might prevent trespass on my property by posting a "no trespassing" sign, erecting a picket fence, stringing up barbed wire, posting an armed guard, or planting lethal explosives around the perimeter of my property. What determines whether any of these coercive actions is justified is whether I have a right to do them, that is, whether my action is consistent with the freedom of everyone, under universal law, and not whether the effect of my doing them is anticipated to affect your interests in a reasonable way, for example, should you decide to trespass on my property. What makes my action right is that it is an exercise of my free choice that is compatible with the freedom of everyone under universal law. You have no rightful complaint against me if you trespass on my land and lose a leg to my land mine: your trespass was not compatible with the freedom of everyone under universal law, while my placement of land mines on my property was. This is not to say that restrictions on land use—perhaps requiring that dangerous land be clearly posted or requiring that the placement of land mines be accompanied by high fences to protect the physical safety of children or those who accidentally trespass—are not possible on Kant's view of right.[26] Instead, the point is about the concept of right itself: most basically, what determines whether something is right is whether it is compatible with the freedom of others under universal law, not how those actions affect others' interests.

The question "How can coercion be morally justified?" may naturally seem to suggest that coercion is a bad thing and that it can only be justified by some more morally weighty countervailing consideration. But this is not the picture of coercion or its justification that Kant presents. Instead, coercion is *any* action that poses a hindrance to the freedom of others, and the only thing that can make such actions rightful is that they can coexist with the freedom of everyone in accordance with universal law. On the Kantian view, right *just is* the authority to coerce,[27] because to say that someone has a right to do something is to say that they are free to do it, *even if* that action coerces others, that is, hinders their freedom.

Kant helpfully illustrates this view of justified coercion with an image from physics. To elaborate slightly on his illustration, we can imagine the domain of rightful external freedom created by universal laws represented by a sphere or defined three-dimensional space, within which an inanimate body (representing the right holder) may move freely, but outside of which it may not move. Simply by moving within its defined space, the body presents an obstacle or constraint to other bodies that would enter that space. If another body enters that space, the first body might repel it simply as a consequence of colliding with it while moving freely within that space, thus causing an equal and opposite reaction.[28] This constraint exists despite the fact that the body floating in the space does not necessarily intend to present an obstacle to other bodies that might enter that space. Merely by occupying and moving within the space, the body poses a constraint or obstacle to other bodies.

Similarly, because each person constrains the freedom of others simply by acting freely in her domain, and they constrain her in the same way, the picture that emerges is one of a continuous "reciprocal and equal coercion."[29] The coercion is equal because the domain of each is carved out under the same universal law, and the coercion occurs merely as an effect of acting freely within that domain. Similarly, the universal law also makes each person equally free at the same time, because although each is constrained by others acting freely within their own domains, each is also free to act without constraint in his or her own rightful domain.

The normative domain of external freedom that is secured to each person under universal law defines the area in which he or she may rightfully move or act. This domain is not reduced by those who enter it in a non-rightful way; the original right holder retains rights over the space, and so retains a right to do anything in that space that she could have done before the infraction, even if this has lethal consequences for the invader. All this can be defined without any appeal to the intentions of either party or the effects on the interests of the party that is rightfully coerced. Rightful action is determined by whether that action can coexist with the external freedom of everyone, in accordance with universal law, and nothing else.

SOLVING THE PROBLEM OF LEGITIMACY?

In chapter 4 I described the main problem of justifying laws and policies as the problem of legitimacy: what makes the exercise of political power morally justified? I argued that any Kantian solution to this problem must explain how coercion can be morally justified, and that it must do so without depending on making persons act morally. It must additionally explain how the government can have a monopoly on the making, interpreting, and enforcing of law without undermining the moral equality of persons. We can now consider the progress Kant's basic account of justified coercion makes toward meeting each of these challenges. I will argue in what follows that Kant's account of justified coercion explains morally justified coercion in the most relevant sense, but not in the more ambitious sense suggested in chapter 4; that his justification does not rely on making persons either directly or indirectly moral; and that he achieves this without undermining equality because his justification is premised in the moral equality of persons. Justifying coercion in the more ambitious sense suggested in chapter 4, and demonstrating that the government's monopoly on the exercise of political power is consistent with the moral equality of persons, are problems that cannot be solved without Kant's account of public right, which will be the topic of chapter 6.

Coercion

I have, so far, described Kant's explanation about how coercion can be morally justified. Coercion is any hindrance to freedom, and is rightful in the case that it does not conflict with the freedom of others under universal law. But Kant's explanation of morally justified coercion may seem to fall short of justifying coercion in the sense we would expect. First, Kant does not seem to justify coercion in the sense that it is usually meant. Coercion is usually defined as an action that is *intended* to frustrate or counteract the voluntary act of another person through the use or threat of force. Kant changes the definition of coercion so as to encompass *any* hindrance to freedom, not just intentional coercion.

Second, it may seem that Kant has changed the question being asked about coercive actions. Instead of showing that coercive acts can be justified vis-à-vis the Categorical Imperative—that is, the moral principles outlined in the *Groundwork*—Kant shows only that they can be justified with respect to the Universal Principle of Right. Consequently, his argument does not seem to provide an answer to the question about how intentional coercion can meet the tests posed by the Formula of Universal Law and the Formula of Humanity. The argument does not show that it is possible to will a maxim involving coercive action, whose end is the frustration of another's ends, as a universal law. And it does not show that coercive actions can ever treat others as ends in themselves, rather than as mere means. All that the argument shows is that it is possible to coerce others in a way that is consistent with their external freedom under universal law. Let us now consider these apparent shortcomings in turn.

The Wrong Definition of Coercion?

First, by defining coercion as *any* hindrance to freedom, Kant makes the concept of coercion unusually expansive. This may seem to call into question whether Kant's argument justifies coercion in the relevant sense for answering the question of political legitimacy.

We can see some of the unusual features of his view by comparing it to a definition given by Beauchamp and Childress. Following an influential discussion by Nozick,[30] they define coercion as an intentional use of a "credible and severe threat of harm or force to control another."[31] Whether a threat is actually coercive, they note, depends on whether it is perceived as both credible and severe and whether the threat is ultimately effective in displacing "a person's self-directed course of action." Coercion, on this account, is also a moralized term because its purpose is to undermine the willingnesss of the person being coerced. Because willingness is a significant feature of autonomy, and there is a prima facie ethical duty to respect the autonomy of rational agents on Beauchamp and Childress's account, coercion is prima facie immoral. So, in contrast to the earlier discussion of Kant's view, this account understands coercion as intentional, effective, and moralized.

Kant's definition of coercion is what might be understood as a rational reconstruction of the concept of coercion. It is not strictly intended to reflect common usage, and Kant does not present it as such. Consequently, it is not strictly a competitor to contemporary theories of coercion that attempt to describe coercion in a way that reflects dominant usage of that term, or that may be offering their own rational reconstruction of the term for different purposes (for example, for the purpose of determining the ethics of decisions made by health care professionals in clinical or research contexts).

Although Kant's definition of coercion may have a different purpose than contemporary accounts, we can compare Kant's understanding of coercion with the one offered by Beauchamp and Childress (and frequently accepted in contemporary accounts of coercion[32]) and see three advantages offered by Kant's concept of coercion when understood as a rational reconstruction for use in political contexts.

First, a central point of difference between the hindrance to freedom and the credible and severe threat accounts is that the latter understands coercion to exist only when one party intends to control the behavior of the other. On Kant's account, coercion is just any hindrance to freedom, whether intended in that way or not. Because Kant defines coercion as *any* action that is a hindrance to freedom, Kant could agree that all "credible and severe threats" are instances of coercion. So, the Kantian account understands intentional threats (and uses of force) as coercion. Insofar as the Kantian account succeeds in justifying hindrances to freedom, he can certainly justify intentional efforts to control others by threats.

Kant's view may seem to include too much in the definition of coercion, by including non-intentional influences as well. But on further reflection, Kant's definition of coercion seems better suited for use in a political theory than does a concept of coercion that relies on the intentions of the actors, because the coercive aspects of governmental actions may often be unintended.

I said earlier that the exercise of political power includes enforcement of laws. An important part of enforcement is the intention to control behavior by the use of threats. Such actions qualify as coercive on both the credible and severe threat account and the hindrance to freedom account. However, on the credible and severe threat account, these threats will only be coercive with respect to the behaviors they intend to produce, because coercion is defined by its intention. Consequently, in cases where threats do not have the intended consequence, the threats are not actually coercive. For example, consider laws that require caregivers to report HIV+ status to officials, that require therapists to report patients communicating intent to harm others to the police, or that require physicians to report teenage pregnancies to parents. Such laws are ostensibly intended to coerce physicians for the purpose of protecting prior partners, potential victims of violence, or parental rights, respectively. However, all three kinds of laws also seem to coerce patients even though though that is not the primary intention behind them: by incentivizing physicians to disclose confidential patient information, the laws also effectively disincentivize patient disclosures and may even cause some patients to forego obtaining care altogether. Although such laws seem to coerce both physicians and patients, on the severe and credible threat account they actually do not coerce patients at all, since the threats were intended only to affect the physicians. Presumably, however, when we evaluate the coercive aspects of enforcement, we are not asking only whether the the *intended effects* are morally justified, but also, what justifies the use of means that may affect a variety of parties in different and often unintended ways. This seems like a problem with the "severe and credible threat" account. In contrast, because the hindrance to freedom account does not regard intentions as an integral part of coercion, it allows us to evaluate any actions involving threats (or other hindrances to freedom) as instances of coercion. The Kantian view allows us to ask, for example, whether laws that unintentionally induce persons to avoid care justifiably coerce them, whereas the credible and severe threat cannot understand those persons as coerced at all in cases where they are not the intended targets of the threats.

Moreover, the credible and severe threat account understands coercion to occur only when effective. This poses several problems for understanding coercion in a political context. Most importantly, coercion on this account can be justified only after the fact because actions that are intended to coerce but do not successfully alter behaviors in the intended way are not instances of coercion at all. When evaluating potential laws and policies, however, we want to know whether the use of certain means—such as threats to imprison or fine—are justified, even if they *do not* effectively control behavior, in some or even most cases. The fact that someone did not comply with my command despite my threat to maim or imprison does not, presumably, directly impact the moral status of my threat. While there are other ways of evaluating the morality of such threats without necessarily calling them coercion, when we ask whether the coercive aspects of laws or policies are morally justified, it seems that what we want is a prospective, rather than retrospective, justification. We want to know whether the means is justified, even if it fails to influence behavior in some or most instances. On the hindrance to freedom account, any hindrance to freedom is coercion, by definition, and the rightfulness or wrongfulness of such actions can be judged prospectively, when judged by the requirement that they be consistent with the freedom of everyone under universal law.

Third, the severe and credible threat view is a moralized one, at least in the context of Beauchamp and Childress's theory. However, a significant problem with moralized theories of coercion becomes especially clear in the context of the question of political legitimacy. This problem is the simple fact that a huge swathe of government activity is coercive, under any definition.[33] The government regularly issues severe and credible threats of harm, intended to control behavior, that actually do succeed in changing the course of individual behaviors. If coercion is moralized, that is prima facie immoral, then this suggests that all these actions stand in need of moral justification, and the wrong of coercion must be outweighed by other moral goods. Such an approach seems cumbersome, especially when applied to paradigmatic cases of justified coercion. For example, neither brandishing a weapon to deter someone who is trying to rob me, nor placing a sign threatening to prosecute trespassers seem to be prima facie wrong at all. We do not think of such paradigmatic cases of coercion as standing in need of justification; we would rather think that any attempt to interfere with these basically justifiable actions would be prima facie wrong, and in need of justification.

On the Kantian view, coercion is not a moralized term, and its moral permissibility cannot be judged until it is placed within the context of freedom under universal law. Credible and severe threats of harm will always count as coercive acts on the Kantian view, and often—although not always—will also count as *wrongful* coercion on the Kantian definition. This is because many "credible and severe threats of harm" involve actions that are not consistent with the external freedom of persons under universal law. For example, paradigmatic cases of coercion involving criminal threats to maim or murder someone who does not act in a preferred way are clear cases of threats to harm that are also wrongful, as in, not consistent with the external freedom of others under universal law.

However, in at least some cases, the Kantian account will find that credible and severe threats of harm, while qualifying as coercion, are not wrong. The reason for this hinges on the vagueness of what it means to "harm." A harm is often understood as a set back to someone's interests. But not all instances of setting back someone's interests are necessarily wrongful. For example, within the context of close economic relationships—such as that between employer and employee—both parties have the ability to set back the others' interests, sometimes severely. The credibility and severity of a threat in such cases—such as a threat from the employer to fire the employee, or a threat from the employee to quit—depends on circumstances of supply and demand surrounding the threat. Although such threats may be coercive on either the hindrance to freedom account or the credible and severe threat account, they are not necessarily wrongful according to the former. On the Kantian account, the ability to form or fail to renew contracts is a basic extension of each party's rightful freedom under universal law. On Beauchamp and Childress's severe and credible threat view, however, threats to dissolve the relationship are presumably prima facie immoral, at least insofar as they are offered to control the other party.

None of this is to say that Beauchamp and Childress's definition of coercion (or other similar contemporary accounts) is *wrong*. Kant's concept of coercion is particularly well-suited, however, as a method for understanding the moral justifiability of political power, and so for presenting a solution to the problem of political legitimacy.

Rightful, Rather than Moral, Coercion

Kant's justification of coercion may seem to be justification with respect to the wrong principle. In chapter 4 we noted the difficulties involved with justifying intentional coercion by the Formula of Universal Law and the Formula of Humanity. The Kantian account of coercion I have offered thus far—basically, that coercion is rightful if and only if it can coexist with the freedom of others under universal law—is an account of the rightfulness of coercion, and not an account about when it is *moral*. For all formulations of the Categorical Imperative, showing that an action is moral requires showing that the action is done for the right reason. This is a higher bar and a more ambitious sense of "morally justified" than showing merely that an action is rightful. This raises the prospect that persons acting coercively—such as those passing and enforcing laws—may act within their rights without acting morally, all things considered.

But on further reflection, the question about whether an action is rightful is the more relevant question for a theory of political legitimacy. This is so for two reasons. First, the morality of a coercive action is not always possible to determine from an external standpoint, and in some cases may be difficult to determine even from a first-person perspective. People have different reasons for doing different things, and their reasons are often opaque to us. For example, imagine a person who allows neighborhood children to take a shortcut across his corner property for many years. Soon after a homeless man begins using the shortcut, the neighbor erects a fence around the border of his property, making trespass impossible (or at least much more difficult). Did he do this for discriminatory reasons? It is difficult to be sure, from an external perspective. Even if he denies doing it for discriminatory reasons, we may not fully believe him. But even if we do not, it does not seem that we can conclude that he is prejudiced against the homeless. After all, morality presumably requires not discriminating based on whether someone has a home, but does not require that persons avoid doing things that might be perceived as discriminatory, despite having other motivations. Any number of reasons could explain why he erected the fence at that time, some of which are presumably morally innocuous. From an external standpoint it is often not possible to determine what motivates someone else.

Moreover, although it is possible that he intentionally deceives us about his motivations in building the fence, it is also conceivable that he thinks his motivations were not discriminatory, even though they actually were. At least some of the time, people tell themselves that they act on reasons other than those actually motivating them. This raises the prospect that we are not always accurate judges of even our own motivations and may not have an accurate understanding of the reasons for an action even from a first-person perspective. As Kant puts it,

> it is absolutely impossible by means of experience to make out with complete certainty a single case in which the maxim of an action otherwise in conformity with duty rested simply on moral grounds and on the representation of one's duty . . . for we like to flatter ourselves by falsely attributing to ourselves a nobler motive, whereas in fact we can never, even by the most strenuous self-examination, get entirely behind our covert incentives.[34]

The epistemic problems associated with judging motives are amplified with respect to laws, because laws are the product of a multitude of actors. There are the constituents who vote a representative into power, based on what they hope that person will do. Even if they agree about what they want from that representative, they may have different motivations for wanting those things. Furthermore, each law is a product of the efforts and votes of a multitude of legislators with different intentions, sometimes in negotiation with the executive branch, and the effect of the laws may be altered either by later judicial interpretation or by choices made in the process of executing the law. If we can't always know the motivations of individuals, the problems are that much harder when it comes to judging the reasons behind such coordinated efforts.

While we are often not epistemically positioned to make an accurate judgment about others' motivations, a judgment about whether an action is rightful—that is, whether it is compatible with the external freedom of everyone under universal law—is possible to determine from either a first- or second-person perspective. As I've argued, this question is about the nature of our external behaviors. It abstracts altogether from the reasons for which a person acts, and so need not rely on motivations that are in many cases unobservable. So, in political contexts a theory about the rightfulness of coercion is more valuable than a theory of the morality of coercion (at least, a Kantian one), because the theory of rightfulness can help us make judgments about the justifiability of coercive actions even when we do not know the motivations behind them.

Second, politics must prioritize concern with the rightfulness rather than the morality of actions because, even when we are able to accurately judge the reasons on which others act, knowing that they act immorally does not necessarily change our rights in relationship to them. For example, suppose in casual conversation my neighbor comments that he put up his fence because he has had "enough of the homeless" and that they should "get a job." Despite his immoral motivations, his action does not clearly change the nature of my duty to respect his rights. He still has a right to a fence on his property, even if it is wrongly motivated. I am no more justified in taking down his fence, for example, than I would be if he had erected it for less discriminatory reasons. The same holds true for immoral pieces of legislation. If a legislature prohibits narcotics, and some members voted for the laws for racist reasons, their motivations are a reason to vote them out of office, but they don't seem in themselves to affect either the legitimacy of the law or the extent of my duty to obey it. Perhaps such laws are illegitimate or perhaps I have no duty to obey them, but regardless, it doesn't seem likely that I need to know the actual motivations of all, most, or even any of the legislators to determine whether they are legitimate or whether I have a duty to obey. What matters is whether the laws themselves are legitimate.

The question that Kant answers here, about the rightfulness of coercion rather than the more ambitious one about whether it is compatible with moral duty, is, I think, the question we should be asking when we ask about the moral justification of political power. What we usually want and need to know is whether political power is exercised justifiably *with respect to us* (or respect to others), not whether it is rightly motivated or whether it was chosen for duty's sake by all those responsible for making, interpreting, and enforcing the law.

Even if the question about whether we have a right to coerce others is more important, from a political perspective, than the question about whether it is moral to do so, it is still important to determine whether it can ever be moral to coerce others. If Kant's political theory shows that we have a right to coerce others under some circumstances, as I have argued, but his moral theory suggests that it is not morally permissible to do so, then we might think that this is a problem for the overall coherence of his practical philosophy. Moreover, from a first-person perspective, it is important to know when our activities are morally justified and not just whether they are compatible with others' rights. Consequently, it is still important to answer the question posed in chapter 4 about whether coercion can ever be morally justified with respect to the Categorical Imperative.[35] I will attempt to answer this question in chapter 6. In sum, however, Kant does show how coercion can be morally justified in the most relevant sense for law and policy—namely, he shows how coercion can be justified with respect to others, regardless of whether it is exercised for the right reasons. Kant's claim is that coercion is rightful if and only if it does not interfere with the external freedom of others under universal law.

Morality

A second challenge for any Kantian account of legitimacy, I argued in chapter 4, is whether it can justify coercion without suggesting, problematically, that coercion can be justified because it enforces morality. We have now explored the basic principles underlying Kant's account of political legitimacy, and this account is sufficient for showing why his account of legitimacy does not rest on enforcing morality.

First, political legitimacy does not rely on enforcing morality because the argument for the most basic principle underlying political legitimacy (the Universal Principle of Right) does not rely on the concept of moral duty. It begins instead with the concept of right, which is concerned only with whether the choice of one can coexist with the external freedom of everyone under universal law. External freedom is a person's freedom to act without interference from the choices of others, and whether a person is "free" in the external sense does not depend on anyone acting morally.

Kant's account of justified coercion, likewise, does not depend on moral principles, such as the formulations of the Categorical Imperative. To say that an action is "coercive" signifies only the fact that it represents a hindrance to another person's choice. Coercion can occur merely as a consequence of acting freely within one's domain of freedom, as defined under universal law. It can be described with the use of spatial metaphors, further emphasizing the independence of externally rightful actions from the reasons for which those actions are performed. The justifiability of a coercive act depends on whether that action is consistent with the freedom of others under universal law, and does not depend at all on whether it makes others act morally, directly or indirectly.

Equality

Finally, in chapter 4 I argued that a Kantian view of political legitimacy must not undermine the moral equality of persons. Because wielding political power involves attempting to exercise a monopoly on making, interpreting, and enforcing laws, this is a particularly difficult challenge.

I will not be able to explain why a government monopoly on political power is consistent with moral equality until the end of the next chapter. But here I can explain the way in which justified coercion is in the most basic case not only consistent with moral equality but is required by it.

Laws, by definition, are about regularity: I am under a law if it is always the case that I must do what it says. The idea of a *universal* law is the idea of a law that holds always, not just for me but for everyone. Universal laws follow from the idea of moral equality. They bind us equally, but also make us equally free. Universal laws of right, as we have seen, simultaneously prescribe duties to each not to interfere with the external freedom of others and prescribe a domain of freedom in which each can act unencumbered by the choices of others. For example, if universal laws require that no one touch anyone else without that person's consent, then they restrict everyone's freedom, but at the same time they create a domain of freedom for each person in which she is free to refuse the touch of others, even if she can still be influenced by the choices of others in other ways. Because the laws are universal, each person is entitled to the same kind of freedom—freedom from being touched without consent—that everyone else is entitled to.

Coercion, as any hindrance to freedom, can be either consistent with the freedom of everyone under universal law, or not consistent with it. If it is consistent with the freedom of everyone, coercion is justified. The possibility of such justified coercion is strictly necessitated by the concept of equality. If you hinder my freedom under universal law, it cannot, morally speaking, change the nature of my freedom: I am still entitled to do the same things, within my domain, that I could if you were not hindering my freedom. This is a consequence of our equal freedom: I am always entitled to act freely within my domain, just as you are in yours. For example, if you decide to drive your car on my lawn, this does not in itself change my freedom to do what I want on my lawn. Since I may move freely on my lawn, I am free to move as I wish on that lawn, even if that means forcibly ejecting you. This authorization to eject is simply a consequence of exercising my lawful freedom. To say that I had no authorization to remove you would be to hold that you could alter my freedom to move as I wish on my lawn by placing yourself there. If that were possible, then we would be unequal: you would be able to alter my freedom by infringing on my domain, but I would not be authorized to do the same to you. So justified coercion is necessitated by equal freedom.

NOTES

1. Readers who would like a more complete defense of Kantian political theory against its competitors might begin by consulting several recent works in this vein, especially Katrin Flikschuh, *Kant and Modern Political Philosophy*, (New York: Cambridge University Press, 2000); Arthur Ripstein, *Force and Freedom: Kant's Legal and Political Philosophy* (Cambridge, Mass.: Harvard University Press, 2009); Louis Philippe Hodgson, "Kant on the Right to Freedom: A Defense," *Ethics* 120, no. 4 (2010).

2. Derk Pereboom, "Kant's Transcendental Arguments," in *The Stanford Encyclopedia of Philosophy*, ed. Edward N. Zalta (2019). https://plato.stanford.edu/archives/spr2019/entries/kant-transcendental/.

3. *Groundwork*, 4:397.

4. The term "right" (German, *Recht*) has three major uses in Kant's *Doctrine of Right* (see Mary Gregor, "Translator's Note on the Text of the Metaphysics of Morals," in *Practical Philosophy*, ed. and trans. Mary J. Gregor, The Cambridge Edition of the Works of Immanuel Kant [New York: Cambridge University Press, 1996], 357–59). It can refer to a right; to a system of laws that is externally given (or a "rightful condition," as I call it below); or to a characteristic of actions that conform to such a system of laws. The concept of right which Kant analyzes at the beginning of the *Doctrine of Right* is fundamental to all three usages. In my discussion here I frequently refer to the familiar idea of *a* right, mostly because that is the sense of the term "right" with which English speakers are familiar. However, the concept of right that Kant uses here is also fundamental to the concepts of a right action and a rightful condition, as we will see momentarily.

5. 6:230.

6. 6:213.

7. 6:325–28. In the case of welfare rights, the need of one party is taken to signify a change in the choices available to that party, as well as the choices available to the other(s) who have an obligation to meet that right. Welfare rights, insofar as they are "rights" at all, must be cashed out in terms of how the needs of one can change the relationship between his choices and the choices of others, under specific circumstances.

8. 6:230.

9. For an account of rights as divided into active and passive freedoms, see Leif Wenar, "Rights," in *The Stanford Encyclopedia of Philosophy*, ed. Edward N. Zalta (2010). http://plato.stanford.edu/archives/fall2010/entries/rights/.

10. The idea that choices can be *free* in the sense of "not determined by inclination," is necessary for any concept of others as morally *or* legally responsible. Otherwise, on Kant's view, people would have only "animal choice." Their actions would be determined entirely by instinct, and it would make no sense to hold them morally or legally accountable. As Kant points out, in both his moral and political philosophy (both parts of the *Metaphysics of Morals*), a "person" is someone capable of authoring "deeds," meaning someone whose "actions can be imputed to him." 6:223.

11. 6:213.

12. 6:214.

13. For a helpful discussion of external freedom as freedom from being "interfered with or impaired by others," see Jennifer K. Uleman, "External Freedom in Kant's "Rechtslehre": Political, Metaphysical," *Philosophy and Phenomenological Research* 68, no. 3 (2004).

14. 6:230.

15. Leif Wenar, "Rights," in *The Stanford Encyclopedia of Philosophy*, ed. Edward N. Zalta (2010).

16. Wesley Newcomb Hohfeld, *Fundamental Legal Conceptions*, ed. W. Cook (New Haven: Yale University Press, 1919).

17. Wenar, "Rights."

18. Claim rights and power rights are adequately illustrated by Kant's discussion of private property and contract, which discuss both how it is possible to own private property and the means for transferring a property right to someone else. Kant explains the fundamental right of his political philosophy—innate right—by saying that each person has a right to do whatever does not conflict with the rights of others (6:238). This is a privilege right, since it asserts the existence of a right to act in ways that others do not have a right against (in Hohfeldian language, the jural correlate is a "no-right"). An immunity exists in the case that others are unable to alter my rights; it is just the opposite of a power right, and so obtains whenever others lack the power to change a status. For example, Kant argues that people lack a power of self-enslavement, since contracts formed with slaves are unenforceable (6:283); if this is correct, they are immune to self-enslavement.

19. Wenar, "Rights."

20. 6:314. For a similar conclusion about the position of Kant with respect to the interest and will theories of rights, see Ripstein, *Force and Freedom: Kant's Legal and Political Philosophy*, 34.

21. 6:230.

22. 6:231.

23. 6:231.

24. According to Beauchamp and Childress, there is a "common tendency in biomedical ethics to use 'coercion' as a broad term of ethical criticism that obscures relevant and distinctive ethical concerns." Tom L. Beauchamp and James F. Childress, *Principles of Biomedical Ethics*, 7th ed. (New York: Oxford University Press, 2013), 138. They complain that bioethicists use the term to include other kinds of moral wrongdoing, such as exploitation. On their view, coercion is a distinct form of wrongdoing. However, the Kantian understanding of coercion differs from both the understanding offered by Beauchamp and Childress and the "common tendency" they criticize, because it is not moralized.

25. 6:231.

26. Such restrictions can't be explained by rights until a later stage of the argument, that is, after the argument for the moral necessity of a civil condition that can conclusively determine what belongs to each. This account will follow in chapter 6.

27. 6:232.

28. 6:232.

29. 6:233.

30. Robert Nozick, "Coercion," in *Philosophy, Science, and Method: Essays in Honor of Ernest Nagel*, ed. Sidney Morgenbesser, Patrick Suppes, and Morton Gabriel White (New York: St. Martin's Press, 1969).

31. Beauchamp and Childress, *Principles of Biomedical Ethics*, 7th ed., 138.

32. Scott Anderson, "Coercion," in *The Stanford Encyclopedia of Philosophy*, ed. Edward N. Zalta (2008). http://plato.stanford.edu/archives/fall2008/entries/coercion/.

33. Beauchamp and Childress seem to admit as much, when they say that "Coercion . . .[is] occasionally justified—infrequently in medicine, more often in public health, and even more often in law enforcement." Beauchamp and Childress, *Principles of Biomedical Ethics*, 7th ed., 139. However, they do not elaborate on this, and nowhere explain what makes coercion justified in any of these cases, even in medicine. Given the extensive role that coercive laws and policies play in the practice of clinical medicine, as described in chapter 2, it seems that Beauchamp and Childress underrate the importance of coercion in medicine here.

34. *Groundwork*, 4:407.

35. To be clear, determining whether the Categorical Imperative can ever permit coercion is not especially important for the plausibility of Kant's political theory taken by itself, which—as we can see, and as has been argued by others before—does not directly depend on the principles of his moral theory. The question is most important if we take both his moral and political philosophy together, as a coherent whole, as Kant seemed to intend. For the argument that Kant's political philosophy can stand independently of his moral philosophy, see Allen W. Wood, "The Final Form of Kant's Practical Philosophy," *Southern Journal of Philosophy* 36 (1997); Thomas W. Pogge, "Is Kant's Rechtslehre Comprehensive?," *The Southern Journal of Philosophy* 36, no. S1 (1998); Ripstein, *Force and Freedom: Kant's Legal and Political Philosophy*, Appendix.

Chapter 6

State Authority and Morally Justifiable Coercion

We have seen how Kant's account of political legitimacy begins. But his account of justified coercion has mixed success in meeting the three challenges from chapter 4, I have argued. His account explains how coercion can be justified with respect to others. It provides this explanation without relying on enforcing morality, and so it avoids the mistakes most bioethics commentators have made when applying Kantian philosophy to issues in bioethics. And his account explains why the authorization to coerce—and so, justified coercion—is not only consistent with moral equality, but necessitated by it.

However, the account offered so far still faces two important problems in meeting the challenges. First, the account of justified coercion does not clearly explain how the government's possession of a *monopoly* on the exercise of political power can be reconciled with moral equality. Second, the account of justified coercion does not explain how it is possible for acts of coercion to be morally justified in the ambitious sense, that is, justified with respect to the various formulations of the Categorical Imperative. Solving these problems is the main agenda for this chapter.

To solve these problems, we will trace—as briefly as possible—the remainder of Kant's account of political legitimacy. I will roughly follow Kant's own division of the argument, beginning with private right, which includes the accounts of innate and acquired right, and then explaining the account of public right that follows from it. Finally, I will argue that Kant's full account of political legitimacy can meet the remaining challenges in a satisfying way.

PRIVATE RIGHT: RIGHTS IN A STATE OF NATURE

On the Kantian account, as we have seen, rights are just freedoms that can coexist with the freedom of everyone, under universal law. But this is vague: what are the universal laws that govern these freedoms? And, what, specifically, can people have rights to?

Kant begins with an account of the rights that we can have in a state of nature, that is, in a condition in which there are no laws or government. The reason for beginning with a state of nature is that his project is to justify the exercise of political power; to do so, he cannot assume the existence of justified political power but must instead show how it could be authorized in the first place. "Private right" is Kant's term for the rights (and associated duties) that persons have even without a government to enforce them.

Innate Right

In chapter 5 I showed how Kant uses his analysis of the concept of right to develop the Universal Principle of Right: "So act externally that the free use of your choice can coexist with the freedom of everyone in accordance with a universal law."[1] The Universal Principle of Right thus defines our duties of right, namely, the duty not to act in ways that infringe on the freedom of others as defined under universal law. From this, Kant develops a principle he calls *innate right*: Freedom (independence from being constrained by another's choice, insofar as it can coexist with the freedom of every other in accordance with a universal law), is the only original right belonging to every man by virtue of his humanity.[2]

Innate right is simply an assertion of the individual right that corresponds to everyone else's duties as outlined in the Universal Principle of Right.[3] Just as persons have duties not to interfere with the freedom of others, so they have a right against others who would interfere with their freedom.

I spoke earlier of right as dividing up normative space into domains, analogous to three-dimensional space; in the principle of innate right, Kant asserts that each individual has a right to act freely within her domain, set aside for her under universal law. This domain is defined negatively by the rights of others, such that any action is right if it does not conflict with the rights of others, under universal law. One consequence of this is, as Kant says, that a person is "authorized to do to others anything that does not in itself diminish what is theirs."[4]

Innate right is innate because of the kind of bodies persons have. Kant mentions that this right is original to persons by virtue of their "humanity." By humanity, Kant understands our rational nature.[5] Rationality is important because it is the necessary condition for the capacity for free choice. Only those who have the capacity for free choice can have rights, since rights are essentially a protected domain for the exercise of free choice. Because rational nature is a feature of the normal adult human body, persons are entitled to freedom innately, as a result of the kind of bodies they possess. Innate right, then, is not something you have to do anything to gain. Instead, it is the necessary consequence of a capacity that results from normal human development. Similarly, it is not something you can sell or give away, since the right is something you have by virtue of your rational nature and subsequent ability to exercise free choice. You can only relinquish innate right by completely destroying the physical body's capacity to maintain a rational nature.

Innate right is the basis for all other rights. It is because persons have an innate right to freedom that they can acquire other rights, such as rights to property, rights to another's performance as specified in a contract, or a right to act as a fiduciary on behalf of another. Enjoying specific rights—freedoms under universal law—is possible only if a person has the relevant capacity to act freely, and the associated right to be free of others in general.[6]

Acquired Right

Possession

Persons can acquire rights to specific things in a state of nature. Acquired rights, in contrast to innate right, are rights that can be obtained and relinquished by choice.

The meaning of a "right to a thing" can be inferred from the concept of right. As we saw earlier, to have a right is just to have a free choice that can coexist with the freedom of everyone under universal law. Right is concerned only with external freedom, as we saw in chapter 5, which is freedom from interference by others. A right to a thing, then, would be the normative ability to use something free of incompatible uses by others. Or, as Kant puts it, I have a right to a thing if "another's use of it without my consent would wrong me."[7] I alone may determine how that thing is used.

Possessing a right to a thing does not merely mean, as Kant points out, that another's use of it wrongs me only in the case that I am currently using or touching it. We do not need a concept of possession to explain this kind of wrong. If I hold an apple in my hand, and another touches it without my consent, the wrongness of the other's action can be explained merely by referring to innate right: by touching the apple, the other person indirectly touched *me*, and so violated my innate right to be free in my person of constraint by others. Instead, possessing a right to a thing means that others would be wrong to use it regardless of whether I am currently physically touching it. It is a right to the thing considered distinctly from its physical relationship to my person.

How is it possible for me to have such a relationship to an object, such that another's use of it would wrong me even though I am not touching it? The argument is a simple one: it is possible for me to have a right to a thing because having such an exclusive relationship to an object *need not* violate the freedom of others under universal law. If the only things that are wrong are things that are not consistent with the freedom of others under universal law, and I am free to do whatever I want so long as it is consistent with the rights of others, then there can be nothing wrong with me possessing something. I have a right to own things simply because no one else has a right against this. Thus the argument goes like this:

Something is wrong if it violates the freedom of others under universal law.

Possession of an object need not violate the freedom of others under universal law.

Therefore, possession of an object need not be wrong.

However, the possibility of possession applies only to objects of choice, that is, objects that can be used in a way that excludes some use by others. This owes to the fact that right is relational. If my use of an object cannot conceivably constrain or otherwise affect another's use of that same thing, or theirs mine, then I cannot have a right to it because the use of it by either of us does not influence the choices available to the other. For example, I may use the sun's energy to grow my garden or to charge a battery with a solar panel. However, I cannot have a right to the sun's energy because another's use of the sun's energy cannot conceivably influence or otherwise detract from my use of the sun's energy. If their use of the sun's energy cannot in principle affect my freedom to use it, then I cannot have a right to the sunlight. Right is concerned with making the free choice of each compatible with the external freedom of all, but in this case, there is no need for laws to make our freedom compatible: our uses of free choice are necessarily compatible, owing to the fact that it is not possible for me to use sunlight in a way that is incompatible with your use of sunlight somewhere else.

On the other hand, it is possible for me to have a right to the airspace above my garden. Another's use of this *would* impact the choices I have: for example, if someone built a large awning that stretched over the top of my property from one end to the other, this would affect the choices I have available to me, such as whether to plant a garden or use a solar panel. But this would be a right to the airspace, which can be used in a way that excludes other uses, and not a right to the sunlight, even though sunlight may be the thing that I want or need.

The kinds of things to which I can have a right can thus change, according to available technologies. In this case, we can imagine someone inventing something like a solar magnet, capable of drawing in the solar energy from surrounding properties. In such a case, their use of the sun's energy could be incompatible with my use, and so could provoke a question about who had the right to the sun's energy. Specific radio frequencies, or the airspace five miles above a nation, similarly, could not be the object of rights claims in Kant's time, but once radios and airplanes were invented, these things could be used in ways incompatible with the freedom of others.

On Kant's account, although rights are restricted to the class of things whose use is potentially incompatible with uses by others, rights can apply to any of the things in this class. In other words, if it is possible to use something in an exclusive way, then it is possible to own it.[8] This owes to the fact that exclusive use of any particular object *need not* be incompatible with the freedom of others. They can be equally free so long as they have the same freedom, to use thing belonging to them free of incompatible uses by others.

To say that ownership of items *need not be* incompatible with the freedom of others suggests that ownership *can be* incompatible with the freedom of others. But this is to assert nothing more than that it is possible for another to have a relationship with that object such that for me to touch it or use it without their consent would be incompatible with their freedom, that is, it would wrong them. In other words, to say that my ownership of an item is incompatible with the freedom of (one or more) others is merely to say that it is they, and not me, who owns the item.

Because rights of ownership are by definition potentially compatible with the rights of others, persons are generally entitled to own things.[9] Conversely, they have a duty not to use things as though they cannot be owned.[10] This duty may seem abstract, and Kant says little to explain it. But this duty effectively rules out certain kinds of normative claims. For example, it rules out any claim that land—either in general, or some specific piece—cannot belong to anyone.[11] While land may currently belong to no one (or, more accurately, may currently belong to everyone[12]), it could in principle belong to *anyone*. Those who would try to prevent someone from enclosing a plot of land and using it as his own may say they do this because no one *can* own it, but in fact, by excluding the other from that land and using force to back up their determinations, they merely advance a competing claim of ownership of the land. If ownership is just the right to determine who will or will not use something, then *any* attempt to exclude others relies on an incipient claim of ownership, even if it is misleadingly cloaked in moral rhetoric about the impossibility of owning the land at all.

Possession and the Problem of Unilateral Imposition of Obligation

Claiming a right to something external in a state of nature poses a serious problem for equality, however.[13] This is because claiming a right to something external necessarily implies that others have a duty not to interfere with that thing. Making a rights claim in a state of nature is essentially claiming the authority to determine the universal laws that bind everyone, because without such universal laws, there can be no rights or duties, only various interferences with the freedom of others. But no one has the authority to unilaterally determine the obligations of others, in this way: if others are equally free under universal law, then I have no more right to obligate them than they do to obligate me.

For example, suppose you claim that you have a right to all the land in the fertile valley floor. You have taken such land on the understanding that if you have a right to that land, others have a right to other land, such as the inhospitable land that is left over on the mountains. By claiming a "right," you imply that your use of the thing in an exclusive way is compatible with the freedom of everyone under universal law, since this is what a right is. But you also impose a duty on me, consequently, not to farm in the fertile valley. Assuming that we are moral equals, there is no non-arbitrary reason why it is you, rather than I, who gets to decide the content of our respective rights and duties.

The way out of this problem initially appears to be that we could agree to secure our individual rights by agreeing to each other's rights. This solution does preserve our moral equality, but it does not succeed in granting either of us a right. A right, as we have said, is a freedom that is compatible with the freedom of *everyone,* under universal law. An agreement between us may preserve our equality relative to each other, but it does not produce a right because our agreement still represents a unilateral imposition of obligation on others.

Possession and the Problem of Unequal Security

There is a second problem with rights claims to external things in a state of nature, and this problem has to do with the kind and degree of the hindrance to freedom that is connected with particular rights claims.

Although using something always presents a hindrance to the freedom of others insofar as it alters their ability to use that same thing, some ways of using things present more of a hindrance to freedom than others. For example, suppose that, in addition to plowing and planting your land in the fertile valley, you have the means to erect a tall stone fence around your garden and hire a small army to protect it. I am poor, and when I am done plowing and planting my land, the only means I have to keep intruders out is to encircle my property with a string tied to small wooden stakes.

Now imagine that you and I have a meeting, in which we reach agreement about the boundaries of our respective gardens. Consequently, neither of us unilaterally imposes duties on the other. Even so, there is a real sense in which our freedom is not equal. You have the ability to violate my freedom with impunity, because my use of my belongings presents almost no hindrance to your use of it. My use does present a hindrance to your freedom, to some extent: you cannot use the land entirely as you would have, had I not been there. If I have planted beans, you may have difficulty removing them all in order to plant corn. Perhaps the irrigation canals I dug present a minor obstacle to your preferred use of my land. On the other hand, your wall and army present a virtually insurmountable obstacle to my use of your land. So, even though we are equals in the sense that we both gave consent to the extent and boundaries of our land, we are not equally free because we do not hinder each other's freedom to the same extent. Since, as we saw in Chapter 5, coercion is just any hindrance to freedom, we can say that we coerce each other very unequally, because we hinder the freedom of each other to very different extents.

Kant explains this problem in terms of assurance: essentially, you have assurance that I will not violate our agreement, because I am not capable of doing so. But I have no assurance that you will not violate it, because it would cost you very little to violate my rights.

Ownership in a state of nature always presents this problem. The ability of each person to hinder the freedom of others to use his or her belongings will be different, both because of inequalities in our native abilities, and also because of the way these differences can be magnified over time by prudence and fortune. Lacking equal assurance, we are not equally free. Our agreement about our respective rights means little if I am, nevertheless, always subject to your inclination about whether to follow it. I must constantly think of ways to protect what is mine; I may even lack incentive to fully develop my land, knowing that the wealthier I am, the more attractive I am as a target of theft or wars of acquisition.

This problem, like the problem of unilateral obligation, can potentially be solved. You might offer me some kind of assurance that you will not attack, by making yourself vulnerable to me in some way. For example, perhaps you give me the keys to your backdoor, or you offer your daughter to me in marriage, in exchange for similar assurances from me. These may be enough to assure me that you will not violate our agreement about the extent of my property. They may effectively make us equally assured about the security of our rights with respect to each other.

However, just as we saw with the problem of unilateral obligation, a merely bilateral solution might solve the problem of equality between us but doesn't fully achieve rights. My rights are secure only if they are secure against *everyone*. Even if I have assurance from you, this makes my possessions secure against only one person. My rights are not secure until I have assurance from everyone that they will be respected.

Rights in a State of Nature Are Provisional

These problems with rights in a state of nature do not undermine the possibility of rights altogether. As we saw, there is nothing inherently wrong with possessing something in a way that excludes others; there is no necessary reason why such possession would be incompatible with the rights of others. The problems of unilateral obligation and unequal security are problems that are, in principle, corrigible. Property rights *could* be compatible with the freedom of everyone under universal law, if everyone consented to them, and if everyone offered everyone else equal assurance that their rights would remain secure.

These problems with rights claims also do not undermine any *actual* rights claims in a state of nature. While they bring up contingent problems we can expect will attend *any* individual rights claims in a state of nature, they do not conclusively demonstrate that any individual rights claim does not obtain. This is because, as we saw earlier, the only way to show that someone lacks an actual right to something is to demonstrate that such a right violates some other person's rightful freedom. But this would be to advance a competing claim about who had a right to determine the uses of that thing. Such competing claims of rights are attended by exactly the same problems as the original assertion of the right—namely, they imply a unilateral imposition of obligation. In the same vein, any attempt to secure such a right against the original rights-claimant would threaten the freedom of others, including the original claimant.

The consequence of this is that persons have rights in a state of nature, but all such rights are only provisional—that is, they are provisional on the eventual correction of the problems of unilateral obligation and unequal security. The claims are rightful provided that they are exercised in a way that anticipates eventual ratification in a civil condition, that is, a condition in which everyone consents to the rights of everyone else, and in which each provides assurance providing for the equal security of those rights.

The Problem with Provisional Rights

In one sense, provisional rights in a state of nature preserve the equal freedom of all. Each person is equally entitled to claim property, to enter into contracts, and to engage in legally significant relationships like marriage or parenthood. Kant outlines a process for acquiring such rights in a state of nature and argues that all three of these kinds of rights are possible in a state of nature.[14] And each person is equally free to enforce rights claims, and to take steps necessary to provide for his own security.

In another sense, however, provisional rights do not preserve the equal freedom of each. They do not solve the problem of unilateral imposition of obligation. In a state of nature there is no agreement about the extent and boundaries of provisional rights. There is, moreover, no agreement about the rules governing how people can alienate or acquire rights to external things. Indeed, no one has an obligation to honor rules or conventions which do not, by themselves, have the authority to bind persons whose equal freedom gives them as much authority to propose or act on new or different rules than those that have taken hold.

Similarly, provisional rights do not solve the problem of unequal security. If the security of my belongings depends on your whim, we are not equally free. Kant says that if others are unwilling to give me assurance that they will respect what is mine, I am entitled to obtain security by making a pre-emptive strike against them.[15] By allowing them to develop or maintain the ability to take what is mine without fear of consequence, I accede to a situation in which we are not equally secure from each other and so not equally free. This "violent" state of affairs exists even if we take everyone to be acting in good faith, because it is a result of the fact that we will inevitably come to different conclusions about the content of our rights and the universal laws that should bind us.[16]

Rights and the Duty to Enter a Civil Condition

Because provisional rights do not fully guarantee my equal freedom under law, I am authorized to take additional measures to preserve that freedom. This includes, in a state of nature, a general right to force others to recognize what is mine and to give me assurance that they will respect my rights. This is, in other words, a right to force others into a civil condition.[17] I do them no wrong by forcing them into a civil condition because I have a right to be free of their independent determinations about the extent and nature of my freedom.

By forcing them into a civil condition, I force them to recognize what is rightfully mine and to give me assurance that they will not infringe on it; likewise, I recognize what is theirs, and give them assurance that I will not infringe on it. Since a civil condition is one in which all agree on a set of laws governing relations between us, and all offer assurance capable of securing the rights of others, in a civil condition our rights are no longer provisional, but conclusive.[18]

My innate right to freedom, then, cannot be fully established except within a civil condition. And the innate right of others is the same. Because they have a right to force me into a civil condition as well, we finally arrive at the postulate of public right: "when you cannot avoid living side by side with all others, you ought to leave the state of nature and proceed with them into a rightful condition."[19] Each person has a duty, then, as well as a right, to establish a civil condition.

PUBLIC RIGHT: RIGHTS IN A CIVIL CONDITION

The nature of the duty to enter a civil condition has important consequences for the features of our life together once we have entered it. Moreover, the features necessitated by this duty can together explain the final aspect of legitimacy that eluded us in chapter 5: together, they can morally justify the government's monopoly on the exercise of political power.

United Will of All

To see how the government's monopoly on political power can be justified, we can begin by looking at the nature of the agreement that is required by the duty to enter a civil condition. Kant calls the idea of such an agreement the "original contract."[20] This original contract represents the united will of all.

The idea that the original contract represents the "will" of all may seem like a misnomer. There is no reason for believing that everyone ever actually *did*, or even *would*, agree to a civil condition. As Kant says, some people may possibly even be happier remaining in a state of nature.[21] How can we understand Kant's claim that the civil condition proceeds from a united will of all, as the product of universal consent, when some clearly have not or likely would not consent?

As Japa Pallikkathayil argues, the idea of a united will can be understood to play a "heuristic" role here,[22] or act as a placeholder that can help us understand how we are authorized to use others. As I argued earlier, the ability to claim a right to property—and even, as I have argued, the ability to make any choice at all—requires the consent of others, if such uses or choices are to occur without unilaterally restricting the innate freedom of others, something which no one has the authority to do. The only way to alter the rights of others without infringing on their innate right to freedom is to have their consent.

However, we are authorized to use others as though they have given this consent, even if they have not, because attaining equal freedom under universal law requires them to enter into an agreement with us about how our innate freedom will be mutually restricted. We need a specific set of laws, and a process for laying down these laws, if either of us is to attain the equal freedom under universal law to which we are entitled. We can, in other words, understand the civil condition as proceeding from the united will of all because we are entitled to act precisely as though everyone has agreed to such a condition. We can say, then, that *for all practical purposes* everyone does consent to the creation of a civil condition and can be used as though they have.[23] Consequently, the civil condition is understood as formed on the basis of an original contract, even though no such contract may exist and, even if one does, it may not be the object of actual universal consent.

Institutions and Processes of the State

The idea that the civil condition is formed by the united will of all also helps to inform the character of the institutions and processes that are established in it. Specifically, because the civil condition is formed by the united will of all, its institutions and processes must be formed so that they can represent this will. This requires establishing a state, independent of any particular or unilateral will, capable of laying down laws determining what belongs to each; enforcing those laws; and judging how to interpret those laws. Kant says that these three functions and the corresponding authorities who perform them "arise necessarily from the idea of a state as such,"[24] but does not explain this in detail. Still, we can reconstruct the argument to some extent.

First, there must be an independent body designated with the authority to set down laws determining the rights and duties of each. The reason for the duty to enter a civil condition is the necessity that persons' freedom be made equal under universal laws. But laws formed by private citizens would essentially defeat the purpose of entering into a civil condition, because they would constitute unilateral imposition of obligations. So, entering into a civil condition carries with it the necessity of an independent body, conceived of as representing the united will of all, that can write rules for the whole political community—it requires, in other words, a legislative authority or "sovereign."

Second, a civil condition must also contain a body that can effectively offer assurance to everyone, on behalf of all, that their rights will be protected. As we have seen, people cannot be equally free if their rights are not equally secure. My rights may be made secure with respect to specific other individuals if they offer me assurance, but I cannot be equally free to everyone unless everyone gives me assurance. Offering assurance can be compatible with the equal freedom of all only if everyone offers everyone else assurance, so that the resulting coercion can be understood as fully reciprocal. Offering such assurance is possible in a civil condition by placing trust in one body that can protect the rights of each while representing the united will of all. This is the basic rationale for an independent executive authority.

And finally, allowing private persons to judge about how the laws apply to their own cases would necessarily produce the same problems of inequality among citizens. The only way to preserve the equal application of law to each is to have an independent body that does not represent any side in a dispute, but represents the people as a whole and can set down a verdict about what the law requires in particular cases. Just as the civil condition requires both a legislator and an executive authority, it also requires someone who can render a verdict about what the law requires in specific cases; otherwise legislation would be rendered empty and enforcement rendered impotent. This is the basic case for a judicial authority.

Whatever the details about how these authorities are institutionalized in a civil condition, the necessity of entering the civil condition demands that some agreement be made about how specific institutions will fulfill these roles, which are necessary for achieving the purposes for which the civil condition was formed. The institutions and processes set down in the civil condition can then be understood as representing the will of the people, with the corresponding right to rule over citizens considered as individuals. This set of institutions and processes that represent the people as a whole constitutes the "state."[25]

State Authority in a Civil Condition

Because persons have a duty to enter a civil condition and subsequently agree to a constitution settling the institutions and processes that can make, enforce, and interpret law, they also have a duty to submit to the laws and judgments of that body. The reason for such a duty follows from the duty to enter a civil condition. Persons must enter a civil condition in order to respect the rights of others. The institutions and processes set up by the original contract can be understood as established by the united will of all: they are the authorities set up to solve the moral problem associated with life in a state of nature. Citizens must be considered to consent to the determinations of these bodies settled in the original contract for the same reason that they must agree to the original contract in the first place: failure to do so would be to violate the rights of others to have their rights conclusively recognized, and to have their freedom ensured under an equal and reciprocal coercion. Citizens may withhold actual consent from these laws by refusing to vote for them, but once laws have been laid down by the legislative authority, they represent the united will of all. Citizens are bound to them whether they actually consented to them or not, because it is their duty to consent to the civil condition and the institutions and processes by which the laws came about. Consequently, on Kant's account, the state is not only legitimate, but it also has authority:[26] it not only has the right to rule, but also imposes a duty to obey.

Although the state's authority is not a function of any individual person's actual consent, actual consent can still play a role in determining the laws of the state. Laws, like the institutions that form them, are considered to proceed from the united and general will of the people because a people must be considered to come together to agree to these laws. Just as a people could never agree to a set of institutions that were not responsive to the actual will of the people, some provision must be made to ensure that the laws and policies of a state reflect the actual united and general will. One way of accomplishing this is through democratic means, and Kant seems to assume that citizens vote on laws and so can alter the laws governing their freedom through the processes set up in the original contract.[27]

The Limits of Legitimacy

The limits of legitimacy are also determined by the idea of the united will of all. To see why, we need merely return to the way in which the argument developed. The argument for the duty to enter a civil condition, as we have seen, is essentially that people must enter it because doing so is necessary for respecting others' innate right to freedom. The civil condition is a product of the united will of all in the sense that each person has a duty to will the civil condition as a consequence of the more general duty not to interfere with the freedom of others.

The purpose of the civil condition, then, is protecting the freedom of each, consistent with the freedom of all. This purpose also defines the limits of the state's authority, however, because any law that cannot be understood as serving the overall purpose of making us equally free is one that no one has a duty to respect and no one has a right to insist on. When testing the legitimacy of individual laws, then, Kant asks whether the laws *could* be the object of a general and united will of all. This question is not an empirical one, about whether it is hypothetically possible for everyone to agree to the laws; after all, people *can* agree to unjust and incoherent arrangements if they want to, and sometimes they do. Instead, asking whether laws could be the object of a united and general will means asking whether everyone could agree to them *for the purpose of protecting their own equal freedom*.[28] As a shortcut to determining whether some law could be legitimate, we can also ask whether each individual person could agree to the laws. If laws do not serve to protect the equal freedom of each individual person within the civil condition, then the law is one that could not be the object of a united will. I will explore how laws can run afoul of this in chapter 8, when I consider what kinds of legal standards for informed consent could be the object of a united and general will.

Objections

The idea that any law is legitimate that a people *could* will for the purpose of establishing equal freedom under universal law has seemed too permissive to some. There are two important points to remember here. First, it may be more restrictive than is originally apparent. While the idea that any law is legitimate if it *could* be willed seems expansive, Kant's view is that people could will to be constrained only by laws that protect their equal freedom. This rules out, as Kant says, all paternalistic laws;[29] laws that constrain freedoms purely in order to maximize economic growth or achieve other forms of collective welfare are similarly laws that cannot be understood as those equal citizens could agree to because they are not ones that they must consent to, insofar as they are not necessary for achieving equal freedom. Similarly, it would rule out use of law for diverse pet projects, hobby horses, or any other ends that are merely unilateral. Such uses of law would make laws the product of a unilateral will rather than a united and general will. The extent to which Kant's view would permit the laws in any country will depend in part on the extent to which the laws are designed around such illegitimate ends.

Second, Kant's approach may be viewed as too permissive because it does not guarantee any specific outcomes, such as economic equality, overall prosperity, or happiness. But such an objection is question-begging. Kant's view is not intended to yield an ideal set of outcomes because he is concerned with what people have rights to do, not what is in their collective interests, however defined. It may be instructive here to consider the differences between Kant's view and John Rawls's influential theory of justice as fairness. Rawls incorporates many elements of Kantian thought, and even argues that the original position can be understood as a "procedural interpretation of Kant's conception of autonomy and the categorical imperative."[30] Despite Kant's influence on his theory, Rawls defines justice in such a way that it excludes Kant's conception of justice from the outset. For Rawls, society is a cooperative venture for mutual advantage, and justice is the set of rules that divide the "benefits and burdens of social cooperation."[31] While Rawls is most often considered as a theorist of fairness, the principles he proposes for fair cooperation assume an overall purpose for society, and the principles he proposes depend in a crucial way on the negotiations of individuals who are interested in maintaining their own interests in things like income, wealth, and social privileges.[32] This understanding of the concept of justice cannot accommodate the Kantian conception of justice, because the Kantian view does not understand justice, in the first place, as oriented toward achieving or dividing benefits. Instead, justice is a relationship between persons, where they are equally free of each other. The foundational disagreement is in part over whether the purpose of political principles is to secure our freedom from each other or whether it is to secure our mutual advantage on fair terms. Kant's political principles can't guarantee happiness or prosperity because persons have no right to force others to provide them with this; we have an innate right to freedom only, and we can force others into a civil society for the purpose of securing that freedom but not for the further purpose of mutual advantage. Whether Kant's theory of legitimacy is too permissive because it allows nonideal outcomes, then, depends on whether Kant's understanding of justice as equal freedom is right or not.

The good, for Kant, is subservient to the right: the well-being of the state consists not in the happiness or welfare of its citizens but rather in the extent to which its constitution conforms to principles of right.[33] Although the laws chosen in a civil condition may succeed in achieving happiness or well-being to various extents, their success in this regard has no direct bearing on their legitimacy. Legitimacy comes, instead, from the role that laws play in making each equally free. Choosing laws that contribute to happiness, subservient to their role in securing equal freedom—that is, choosing prudent standards for achieving equal freedom—is the prerogative of the electorate, and ensuring the good of the political community over all is something that must, ultimately, be understood as the moral[34] (but not political) duty of individual private persons. A democratically elected government, representing the united will of all, makes it possible for a people to select laws that will further their happiness, so long as the ultimate purpose of those laws is not happiness but the protection of equal freedom.

SATISFYING THE CHALLENGES

In chapter 5, I argued that Kant's account of justified coercion goes some distance toward solving the problem of political legitimacy in a way that satisfies the three challenges of chapter 4. But two problems remained outstanding.

Moral Equality and the Exercise of Political Power

First is the problem of moral equality. I argued in chapter 5 that Kant's account of justified coercion explains why coercion itself is required by moral equality. If you act as a hindrance to my rightful freedom—in other words, if you wrongfully coerce me—the only way of preserving my equality with you is if I can act as a hindrance to your hindrance of my freedom, which is to say, if I can coerce you in return. If you could hinder my rightful freedom without consequence, then you would be able to affect my freedom in a way that I could not affect yours, and we would be unequal. So a right to coerce is required by equality. However, an important problem remains. Even if this explains a general right to coerce, it does not yet explain how the government can legitimately claim a monopoly on the exercise of political power.

We are now able to answer that question. The duty to enter a civil condition is ultimately a consequence of the principle of innate right. If people are entitled to freedom, consistent with the freedom of others under universal law, then they have both a duty and a right to lay down a law that can settle the nature and extent of that freedom—the domain of their rights—in coordination with others who can affect that freedom. The obligation to enter a civil condition carries with it a duty to set up institutions or processes for laying down the laws stipulating what belongs to each by right, offering assurance that each person will act only within their rightful domain of freedom, and judging the application of laws in cases of dispute. It requires, in other words, the creation of a state. The state must, ex hypothesi, represent the people as a whole (a united and general will) and not a unilateral will, because the state is conceived as formed under the agreement made by all the people to give up their lawless freedom, and take it back "undiminished,"[35] as freedom under universal law. They must enter this condition precisely because they lack, individually and severally, the authority to unilaterally impose their will on others. The state must consequently have a monopoly on the making, enforcing, and interpreting of law, because rights claims outside a civil condition, that is, a condition characterized by lack of the rule of a state endowed with these powers, is merely unilateral imposition of law on others equally entitled to freedom. This answers the problem of legitimacy, then, insofar as it explains how the exercise of political power can be morally justified. Not only is the explanation not at odds with the idea of fundamental moral equality, it is actually premised on it. It is only because people are fundamentally morally equal that the need for a state with a monopoly on these powers ever arises.

Coercion under the Categorical Imperative

The second problem is the problem of justifying coercion with respect to the Categorical Imperative. Although I explained in chapter 5 how coercion could be morally justified in one sense—justified in the sense that it is consistent with the rights of others—I admitted that it was not yet demonstrated that coercion could ever be morally justified in a more ambitious sense, that is, with respect to the Categorical Imperative. Justifying coercion under the Categorical Imperative involves more than merely demonstrating that a coercive act does not violate the rights of others. The formulations of the

Categorical Imperative are instead designed to test the reasons for which an action is done: for example, whether the reason for the action is a coherent use of practical reason or if it produces a contradiction, and whether the action is done not just in conformity with duty, but rather, for duty's sake. As Korsgaard has argued, it seems that coercion is the epitome of the kind of action that cannot be justified by the Categorical Imperative, particularly the Formula of Humanity.[36] Coercion always aims to make another person do something that is contrary to their will. However, if coercion cannot be justified with respect to the Formula of Humanity, then we might have to conclude that the coercive enforcement of law is always immoral, even if it is consistent with the rights of others. A Kantian political philosophy should ideally solve the problem of political legitimacy in a way that makes coercive acts of the kind committed by the government at least potentially justifiable in light of the Formula of Humanity.

Kant himself does not directly explain how coercive acts can be moral, but his account of legitimacy does, I think, contain the resources to explain how coercion could be morally justified in the ambitious sense. However, I want to note at this point that we will have to change the question slightly. I have asked whether coercive actions of the kind routinely performed by governments can be morally justified, but no Kantian argument can show that coercive actions in general—or some subset of them—*are* morally justified. At best, a Kantian argument can show that some particular action performed on the basis of some particular end is justified, and thus that actions of that type are potentially justifiable. This owes to the fact that, as we saw in chapter 4, actually morally justified actions are those done *for the right reasons*, that is, for duty's sake. Consequently, instead of asking whether it is possible that coercive laws are morally *justified* with respect to the Categorical Imperative, we must instead assess whether enforcement of coercive laws is morally *justifiable* with respect to the Categorical Imperative. By asking whether a class of actions (in this case, coercive government laws) is morally justifiable, I mean to ask whether it is possible that actions belonging to this class can ever be morally justified, without trying to show that any of them actually are.

I will argue that coercive laws can be morally justifiable when judged with respect to the Categorical Imperative, specifically the Formula of Humanity.[37] In this section I will explain how Kant's concept of right, and the specific rights that follow from it within a civil condition, can be used to mark the distinction between actions that necessarily *use* persons in some way, and those that need not, and can be understood instead as merely *affecting* them. Then, I will argue that actions that violate the rights of others *use* them in a morally significant way and so always fail the test of the Formula of Humanity. Actions that do not violate their rights, however, can be understood as merely *affecting* them. Instances of rightful coercion fall into this latter category and so can, in some cases, pass the test imposed by the Formula of Humanity.[38]

Using and Affecting

The imperative in the Formula of Humanity commands: "So act that you use humanity, whether in your own person or in the person of any other, always at the same time as an end, never merely as a means."[39] The formula requires that when we use a person in some way, we make sure we use that person as an end, and not merely as a means. However, before we can ask whether we use a person as a mere means, we must know whether we are using a person at all. When do I *use* a person in some way or another? It seems obvious that I use you in some way if I do surgery on you without your consent, for example. If I physically touch you, it might seem that I am using you in some way. Or, perhaps I ask to borrow money from you knowing that I will not repay it, much like Kant's case of the lying promisor, who lies about his intention to repay a loan so that a creditor will give it to him.[40] Kant says that the lying promisor uses his creditor as a mere means. So, according to Kant, in such a case I would use you in some way, even though I do not physically touch you. Or, perhaps I avoid lying to you about my intentions to use your money, and instead just steal it. In that case as well, although I have not physically touched you, it seems that I use you as a mere means. I take your money in this case without even a pretense of getting your permission, most likely because I know you will not agree to my taking it. Although I do not directly touch you or even speak to you, it seems that I have used you in some way.

I want to focus on the third case, because I think it is the most interesting. Why should stealing from you be a case of using *you*, rather than a case of just using the money or goods that I steal? At first glance, it may seem that it is using *you* because it is using something that you own. And I think that is close to the truth. But the difficulty is explaining why. Why is using something that belongs to someone using that person rather than just using stuff that they own?

We might think that when I use what belongs to you, I affect you—your place in the world, your overall prospects or position in life—in an important way, and do so for my own ends. But affecting someone in an important way, for my own ends, does not always seem necessarily to be using that person. Suppose, for example, that you manufacture an important pharmaceutical and make your living in that way. I invent a new process that allows me to make the same drug for cheaper. I decide to begin manufacturing the drug, largely on the grounds that I know that I can sell it for less than you can, while still selling it for a high enough price that my expected profits will make it worthwhile for me. By capturing some or most of your customer base, I can make a living.

In this case, just as in the theft case, I am affecting you in an important way. I know that my lower prices will mean my sales cut into your market share: it will either reduce your sales or, potentially, put you out of business. This affects what is already yours—not just what you might have in the future—because my entry into the market will undercut your ability to sell the drug and so will immediately reduce the value of your company. My superior production methods might even make your machines obsolete and so nearly worthless.

Also, note that in this case I affect you in some way for my own ends, and I do so in much the same way that I did in the theft case. I do not (or at least, need not) make this decision *so that* you will go out of business, just as when I steal from you I need not do it *so that* you will lose the amount that I steal. Instead, in both cases, I am driven primarily by my own desire for profit. In both cases, the effect on you is a side effect—foreseen, certainly—of my primary intention. If my theft of your belongings uses you because it affects what belongs to you for my own ends, then it seems as though my action in the drug innovator case is also an instance of using you in some way.

The ethical standard Kant proposes for actions that use someone in some way is that they must use the other as an *end* and never merely as a means. As I discussed in chapter 4, Kant explains what it means to use someone as a mere means: an action necessarily uses another as a mere means if he "cannot possibly assent to it" and if he "cannot contain the end of this action in himself."[41] In cases of stealing, much like cases of lying, the problem would seem to be that it is not possible for the victim to "contain the end of this action in himself." A person cannot assent to being stolen from, precisely because assent renders the subsequent taking a gift, rather than a theft. In cases of theft, the thief steals precisely because he anticipates that his victim will not assent to letting him have it. Even so, in theory I could obtain the money from you without using you as a mere means if I simply asked for permission first and obtained it. By doing so, I use you as an end because I ensure that my actions are consistent with your ends.

But, if this ethical standard is applied to the case of the drug innovator, it produces counterintuitive results. Do I need to ask for your assent before I begin manufacturing and selling the same drug for a lower price? If I do, you will almost certainly refuse to give it. You presumably have no reason to allow a competitor to undersell you and reduce your share of business. I likely use you in a way to which you would *not* assent, even if it is not logically impossible that you could assent. Consider also that any significant action within a market is likely to have multiple such effects: I do not merely affect you my main competitor, but possibly a whole range of competitors, the supply chains on which they depend, and the arrangements they have with distributors, not to mention the effects on consumers and investors. Indeed, in a globalized economy I am likely to have some effect on much of the world, even if in many cases this effect is small or does not represent a harm.

It does not seem plausible that I need to obtain the assent of either you (my competitor) or any of the myriad persons my actions will likely affect, just because my action is an intentional one that I can foresee will affect them in a way that will accomplish my purposes. There is some morally significant difference between stealing and underselling a competitor, such that I need to get assent to borrow money but not to undersell a competitor (or to affect others within a market). Intuitively it seems that I use the victim of theft merely as a means if I take her money without first obtaining her assent, but I do not use a competitor merely as a means if I undersell her without first obtaining assent. This difference seems to persist even if we imagine that the amount I steal is relatively small and my victim is relatively rich, while the loss I inflict on my competitor is large, and she cannot afford it. What can account for this difference?

Rights as a Morally Significant Distinction

In order to plausibly apply the Formula of Humanity, Kant needs a way of distinguishing between actions that *use* others in some way, and so require determining whether they use those others as ends or mere means, such as in the case of theft, or the case of the lying promisor; and actions that merely *affect* others, and for which their assent is not strictly necessary, as in the underselling actions of the drug innovator. Without such an account, Kant cannot explain why we do not need the assent of competitors in cases like drug innovator. And, without such an account we might worry that Kant cannot clearly even explain why taking someone's money without their assent would constitute using them as a mere means: the person who steals this money can always claim that they merely *affected* the person from whom they took the money, and did not necessarily use that person as a mere means. Kant does not provide a rubric in the *Groundwork* to distinguish between using someone and merely affecting them. However, the account of right provided in the *Doctrine of Right* can help to solve this problem.

Kant seems to have gained appreciation for the difference between using someone in some way and merely affecting them by the time that he wrote the *Doctrine of Right*. As we have seen, there he points out that literally *any* choice I make affects others and can be conceived of as a hindrance to their freedom. Stealing from someone is hindering their freedom. Lying to someone about my intention to repay her is a hindrance to her freedom as well. So is setting up a new business and underselling a competitor. Even walking to my mailbox to check the mail is a hindrance to freedom, insofar as it makes this path less available to others who would use it at the same time. Kant solves this problem by arguing that we do not have a right to freedom *simpliciter*: instead, we have a right to freedom that can coexist with the freedom of others under universal law. This creates a domain of freedom for each person, within which they have a right to be free of specified kinds of interference.

This distinction between actions that infringe on your rightful freedom and actions that infringe on your freedom *simpliciter* can also be used to distinguish between actions that necessarily use you in some way and actions that can be understood as merely affecting you. Roughly, we have seen, your domain of freedom includes at least your body and your property. If my action affects your body or your property (or anything else belonging to you) in a way against which you have a right, then I do not merely affect you, but necessarily use you in some way.

Providing a full account about why doing something against which you have a right necessarily uses *you* in some way would take us deep into Kantian normative ethics, and so is beyond the scope of our discussion here.[42] For now, I think it is sufficient to say that Kant strictly needs an account of the distinction between actions that necessarily use others in some way and those that merely affect them. This is because, as becomes clear in the *Doctrine of Right*, *all* of our actions affect others, and it is not plausible that I should have to understand all of my actions as necessarily using others in some way, because this would effectively mean I must gain the assent of others before I do *anything*. Kant needs an account of the distinction between actions that necessarily use others in some way and so must be morally justified, and those that merely affect them and so do not need such justification; and rights can be used to mark this distinction. Let us assume that rights can mark this distinction, then, and examine the implications of such a distinction.

If I necessarily use you in some way when I act in ways against which you have rights, then your assent—or let us call it *consent* now, since that is the better term for explaining what you do when you allow me to do something that would otherwise violate your rights—would be strictly necessary[43] in such cases if I am to avoid to using you as mere means. I must ensure that my action not only achieves my ends, but that it is also consistent with yours, and I must do this by obtaining consent. If I do not obtain your consent, then I use you as a mere means even if you would have consented to my action: my end of using you in some way before you have given actual consent is an end that you could not coherently contain in yourself (if you did, then you would, by definition, already have given consent). So in these cases, where I act in ways against which you have rights, I must obtain consent. Further, I cannot do any of the things that would make your consent impossible, such as use force, coercion, or fraud. By making consent impossible I would use you in a way to which you could not possibly assent: my end in undermining the voluntariness of your consent would be one you cannot possibly share or "contain in yourself."[44]

In other cases, however, where I affect you in a way against which you do not have a right, I do not *necessarily* use you in some way at all, and so my action does not strictly require your assent. Such cases include rightful uses of my freedom where your assent is not only not required, but also often not even relevant. For example, if I begin producing a drug and undersell you, not only do I not need your assent, but your assent is not relevant at all, despite the fact that I may put you out of business. If I put up a fence around my property, I affect your ability to walk across it. Even if I do this in order to *stop* you in particular from walking across my property, I need not understand myself as doing something to you, or using you in some way; in fact, the best way of describing what I am doing may be that I am protecting my property from trespass, or perhaps keeping my lawn pristine, or making my home and family more secure. My action affects you but it does not use you, so I do not need your assent to put up the fence. If you find out about my plan to erect a fence and inform me that you withhold your assent, it doesn't mean that if I put up the fence anyway, I have used you as a mere means to my ends: your ends with respect to a fence on my property are simply not relevant.

Kantian Coercion and the Formula of Humanity

If we take rights as the distinction between actions that necessarily use others and those that may merely affect them, then we are now in a position to give an account of morally justifiable coercion—that is, justifiable in the ambitious sense, justifiable with respect to the Formula of Humanity. First I will show how coercion in the Kantian sense can pass the test imposed by the Formula of Humanity, and then, argue that coercion as defined by the credible and severe threat account can pass the test in much the same way.

Coercion, in the sense that Kant uses the term, is any action that is a hindrance to freedom. Kant argues that coercion comes in two forms: it can be a hindrance to freedom in accordance with universal laws, in which case it is wrong; or it can be compatible with such freedom, in which case it is right. To say that coercion is rightful is not to say that it is justifiable according to the Categorical Imperative, as we have noted, but only that it is justified with respect to the rights of others.

However, if we take persons' rights as the distinction between actions that necessarily use them in some way and those that merely affect them, then we can see why wrongful coercion will always fail the test imposed by the Formula of Humanity. To wrongfully coerce someone is to act in a way against which they have rights. Such actions can only be made rightful if the coerced person gives consent. To act in a way against which they have rights is also, as I have said, to *use* them in a particular way, such that their consent is required if I am to use them as an end rather than a mere means. In cases where I act in ways inconsistent with others' rights without first obtaining consent, then, I will also use them as a mere means. In such cases I violate both the Universal Principle of Right and the Formula of Humanity at the same time.[45]

On the other hand, acting in a way that *is* consistent with others' rightful freedom is also coercive, in the Kantian sense, because this also serves as a hindrance to their freedom. But such actions are just extensions of my own rightful freedom. I am broadly authorized to do anything that does not conflict with their rights. Any use of freedom, I argued, is coercive in this sense, but not in a wrongful way: as Kant puts it, a rightful condition just is one characterized by an equal and reciprocal coercion. Simply by exercising my rightful freedom—putting up a fence around my yard, checking my mail, bringing a drug to market—I coerce others. If I do these things in a way that can coexist with the freedom of others under universal law, I coerce others but do not wrong them.

Such coercive actions are not only rightful but may also be moral. If I am not necessarily using others in some way when I do things like put up a fence around my yard, then the fact that it is not their end that I put up the fence, or that they may withhold assent, is not enough to make it wrong. Since my action can be understood as something I do for some other purpose, that affects them but does not necessarily *use* them, their lack of assent to the fence does not show that I have used them as a mere means by erecting it. I haven't obviously used them in any way at all such that I would need to consider whether my action is compatible with their ends. Putting up a fence is coercive, on Kant's account, because it hinders freedom. But in this case, the coercive action can be morally justifiable because it does not use the other as a mere means. In fact, it may not use the other in any way at all. So, this explains how coercive actions (coercion on Kant's view, as any hindrance to freedom) need not necessarily use others as mere means, even though they do not assent to them.

Mundane uses of coercion—putting up a fence around my property, for example—are, as we have seen, not qualitatively different from those that involve more severe threats or uses of force. The same rationale that allows me to put up a fence around my property—namely, it is a rightful exercise of my equal freedom—allows me to post a warning that I will shoot trespassers, and even authorizes me to use deadly force in the case that someone trespasses.[46] Such actions are coercive, but they are a hindrance to a hindrance to freedom under universal law, and so are authorized. If they were not, then others could unilaterally affect my equal freedom just by violating my rights;

they could affect my right to shoot my gun on my property, for example, simply by walking there. This would make us unequal.

Such uses of freedom, even the use of lethal force, need not be understood as using others as mere means, for the same reasons that putting up a fence around a property does not use others as a mere means. It is only when we act in ways violating the rights of others that we must be understood as using them in some way. On other occasions, it is possible to understand our actions as affecting, but not using, them in a way that requires moral justification, or would require their assent. Shooting trespassers can be understood as a byproduct, a necessary consequence, of pursuing ends that are otherwise permissible or even morally required.[47] In this way, shooting a trespasser may have a deadly effect on that person, but need not be understood as an action that uses them in some way and so requires their assent. I may be shooting them in order to protect my life or other rights; in that case, their death can be understood as a foreseeable consequence of my action protecting myself, rather than a case where I use them.

This does not mean that shooting a trespasser will *necessarily* be morally justifiable. Just because an action need not use another as a mere means does not mean that it actually does not use the other as a mere means.[48] This is because actions that do not violate others' rights may still use them as a mere means; in these cases, whether I use another as a mere means depends on the quality of my maxim when I act. For example, it may be just as easy for me to protect my rights against trespassers by erecting a fence or posting signs as it is to do so by posting an armed guard. Or, perhaps the trespassers can be just as easily ejected by calling the police or asking them politely to leave. I may make my goal to use some person as a mere means to my end, even though my actions don't strictly entail that I am doing so. Similarly, even though I have every right to set up a business that effectively reduces the profits of my competitors, I may still *use* them as a mere means insofar as I set up the business expressly for the purpose of putting them out of business (rather than, for example, to secure a profit). On the Kantian account, I have an imperfect duty to seek the happiness of others, and to support their morally permissible ends. Acting in a way specifically designed to frustrate their goals would violate these requirements. So even though rightful actions need not use others as a mere means, some rightful actions will nevertheless use others as a mere means. What I have argued is that actions that violate the rights of others necessarily use others as a mere means, while actions that do not violate their rights may not.

The Moral Permissibility of Legal Coercion

As we saw earlier in this chapter, a person's rights in a civil condition are not simply those rights they may think are compatible with the freedom of everyone under universal law. Instead, in a civil condition each person's rights are laid down through processes and institutions that they agree to in the original contract, as the determination of a united will. The enforcement of such laws then is rightful coercion, where coercion is understood in the Kantian sense as a hindrance to a hindrance to freedom. Not only does the enforcement of laws not violate the rights of those that are coerced, but submission to such coercion is a duty of right incumbent on everyone.

Because enforcement of laws is rightful coercion, it does not violate persons' rights at all. They have no right to give or withhold consent to the enforcement of laws within a civil condition. While it is possible to use someone as a mere means even when we act in ways that do not violate their rights, such actions *need* not do so; and so, enforcement of laws need not ever necessarily be considered to use those who are the targets of the enforcement as a mere means. Enforcement of legitimate laws affects persons without necessarily using them. The coercive enforcement of a law need not then be understood as an action directed at the persons who are coerced, but can instead be understood as actions directed at protecting the rights of others. Consequently, whether persons assent to being forced to comply with legitimate laws is not a question that we need to ask at all. Coercive enforcement of laws passes the test in the Formula of Humanity because this enforcement can affect persons without using them. Lawful apprehension of a criminal thus requires his assent no more than erecting a fence to keep him out of property he does not own. In both cases the criminal is affected by the rightful actions of others but is not necessarily used in some way that makes him a mere means.

This conclusion applies in the same way even if we understand "coercion" in a more restrictive way than that intended by Kant (indeed, it can apply precisely because the Kantian definition of coercion is so expansive). If we follow more recent authors in understanding coercion as the intentional use of a "credible and severe threat of harm or force to control another,"[49] coercive laws can still pass the test imposed by the Formula of Humanity. Coercive laws regularly threaten fines, imprisonment, or worse in the case that someone breaks the law. These are great harms. But in the case that such harms are threatened to protect the rights of others, and they only threaten harm in the case that someone violates someone else's rights, the threats of punishment are compatible with the rights of wrongdoers and so need not be understood as using them in a way that runs afoul of the Formula of Humanity. They may not assent to such coercive measures, but their assent is not relevant in these cases precisely because enforcement does not violate their rights.

Nor can it be argued against such coercive measures that they make assent impossible by taking away the ability of the wrongdoer to give a meaningful, voluntary assent to compliance with the law—to say, in other words, that the wrongdoer could not assent to the coercive means or could not contain the end of the coercive means in herself. Since forcing her to comply with a law does not use her as a mere means, *threatening* to use force against her also does not use her as a mere means. Thus, rightful coercion—whether in a state of nature or in a civil condition, whether exercised by citizens acting within their legal rights or by officials enforcing laws, and whether understood according to the expansive definition set forth by Kant or in the narrower contemporary sense—can pass the test imposed by the Formula of Humanity because it affects those coerced without necessarily using them in a way that would require their assent.

Rights Are Necessary for Applying the Formula of Humanity

Finally, we can see the importance of the account of right for applying the Formula of Humanity. Without the account of right, it is not clear how to determine when an action uses someone in a way that needs to be compatible with their ends, and when an action merely affects someone in a way in which their ends are not directly relevant. The concept of right can make this clear, I have argued, and can also subsequently determine when coercive actions are justifiable and when they use others in a way to which they could not agree.

Rights would not be able to help us determine when coercion violates the Formula of Humanity if the concept of right or the principles of right that follow from it (such as the Universal Principle of Right and innate right) were derived from the Formula of Humanity, as some authors have argued.[50] If principles of right were derived from the Formula of Humanity, then they would just be a special case of the requirement that we use others as ends, rather than mere means; they would not be able to give us additional information about when our actions use others versus when our actions merely affect them. This constitutes a further reason, in addition to those presented in chapter 5, for thinking that the concept of right and the theory of right that is built on it are independent in an important sense from Kant's moral philosophy. It is also another reason for thinking that political philosophy is integral to bioethics. Insofar as applying moral principles (like the Formula of Humanity) to concrete cases depends on a prior conception of rights; and a conception of rights depends on political philosophy; then applying moral principles to cases will depend on political philosophy.

NOTES

1. 6:231.
2. 6:237.
3. The right he asserts here is analytically equivalent to the duties outlined in the Universal Principle of Right. All that Kant adds in his definition of innate right is the idea it is the "only original right" that persons have.
4. 6:238.
5. *Groundwork*, 4:437
6. On Kant's view, children (and so presumably also severely mentally disabled persons) are still free beings, in some sense (6:280), albeit ones who are not capable of taking care of themselves. They have against their parents an innate right to care and education, because the parents brought the child into the world at their own initiative. Although children are possessed of innate right because of their incipient freedom, they are not capable of exercising their rights until they are independent. Before emancipation, their parents have essentially status rights with respect to them, which Kant calls "a right to a person akin to a right to a thing."
7. 6:246.
8. 6:246.
9. Although it may at first appear that Kant needs a further argument showing that rights of possession are not only possible but also necessary, he actually does not. If ownership rights are normatively or conceptually possible—meaning only that they can potentially coexist with the freedom of others under universal law—then any actual ownership claims are in principle plausible. The only way of decisively refuting such a claim would be to assert that ownership was incompatible with the right of some specific person—which would, in effect, be to mount a competing claim about ownership.
10. The Postulate of Practical Reason with Regard to Rights: "act towards others so that what is external (usable) could also become someone's." 6:252.
11. It may be directed specifically against Rousseau's claim, that "The first man, who, after enclosing a piece of ground, took it into his head to say, 'This is mine,' and found people simple enough to believe him, was the true founder of civil society. How many crimes, how many wars, how many murders, how many misfortunes and horrors, would that man have saved the human species, who pulling up the stakes or filling up the ditches should have cried to his fellows: Be sure not to listen to this imposter; you are lost, if you forget that the fruits of the earth belong equally to us all, and the earth itself to nobody!" Jean-Jacques Rousseau, *A Discourse Upon the Origin and the Foundation of Inequality among Mankind* (New York: Bartleby.com, 2001), http://bartleby.com/34/3/.
12. On Kant's account, unowned property is understood as property that is subject to original common ownership (6:262). To say that a person has not succeeded in original acquisition of property is, in essence, to advance the claim that the property is still owned communally by everyone.
13. My account of the problem of unilateral imposition of obligation is influenced in part by Ripstein's illuminating discussion of "Three Defects in a State

of Nature." See Arthur Ripstein, *Force and Freedom: Kant's Legal and Political Philosophy*,(Cambridge, Mass.: Harvard University Press, 2009), Ch. 6.

14. *Doctrine of Right*, Chapter II.

15. 6:307.

16. 6:312.

17. 6:264, 6:312.

18. 6:256–57.

19. 6:307.

20. 6:315. Because this agreement is one that is morally required within a state of nature, it is best understood as a moral ideal that should structure our political life, not a particular historical contract.

21. 6:318.

22. Japa Pallikkathayil, "Deriving Morality from Politics: Rethinking the Formula of Humanity," *Ethics* 121, no. 1 (2010): 141. The idea of a "heuristic" is useful because it approximates Kant's understanding of an "idea of reason"—a truth that we must assume in order to make sense of other concepts, such as the idea of rightful action, in the first place.

23. Onora O'Neill argues that consent to the civil condition is rationally required. See Onora O'Neill, "Kant and the Social Contract Tradition," in *Kant Actuel: Hommage À Pierre Laberge*, ed. François Duchesneau, Claude Piché, and Guy Lafrance (Montréal: Bellarmin, 2000).

24. 6:315.

25. 6:311.

26. Authority is best understood as encompassing both legitimacy (as a morally justified monopoly on the exercise of political power, or a "right to rule") *and* a corresponding obligation to obey. See Michael Huemer, *The Problem of Political Authority: An Examination of the Right to Coerce and the Duty to Obey*, (New York: Palgrave Macmillan, 2013), 42.

27. 6:341. However, Luke Davies argues that Kant does not suggest here that governments must be elected democratically, but only that they must be republican. See Luke J Davies, "Kant on Welfare: Five Unsuccessful Defences," *Kantian Review* 25, no. 1 (2020). Either way, Kant clearly thinks that government institutions are supposed to represent the actual will of the people in some respect.

28. Onora O'Neill calls this "modal consent," and gives a helpful discussion of the ways in which it differs from both actual and hypothetical consent. See O'Neill, "Kant and the Social Contract Tradition."

29. 6:317.

30. John Rawls, *A Theory of Justice* (Cambridge, Massachusetts: Belknap Press of Harvard University Press, 1971), 256–57.

31. Rawls, *A Theory of Justice*, 4.

32. In the original position, individuals are assumed to not take an interest in the affairs of others; in this sense they are "mutually disinterested," and they assume that their ends may be mutually opposed. Rawls, *A Theory of Justice*, 13–14. In this way, Rawls designs society around what Kant might call a set of "hypothetical imperatives." Kant scrupulously avoids the use of principles that assume discretionary ends

such as those assumed by Rawls, in part because he recognized that such imperatives cannot be universally binding because the ends on which they are based are not universally shared.

33. 6:318.

34. On Kant's account, one of two ends that are also moral duties is the "happiness of others" (*Doctrine of Virtue*, 6:385). However, this duty does not appear in his political philosophy, because having such an end (indeed, having any end at all) is not something that persons can be forced to do.

35. 6:316.

36. Christine Korsgaard, "The Right to Lie: Kant on Dealing with Evil," *Philosophy and Public Affairs* 15, no. 4 (1986).

37. I focus on the Formula of Humanity in part because it is (according to Korsgaard) more difficult to justify coercion on the basis of this formulation than on the basis of the Formula of Universal Law.

38. The following account is similar in some ways to one offered by Japa Pallikkathayil. The principal difference between our accounts is that I argue that rights are necessary for distinguishing between cases that necessarily use someone and those that do not. On her account, rights distinguish between cases of wrongful use (cases where someone is used as a mere means) and those that do not. On both of our accounts, cases of violating someone's rights will be cases in which others are used as a mere means. However, on her account violating someone's right (or doing one of three other things) will be both necessary and sufficient for violating someone's rights. On my account, violating someone's rights is sufficient but not necessary for using someone as a mere means. I explain the difference in note 48. Although my account was conceived independently of hers, her essay has no doubt influenced the way in which I have approached the question. See Pallikkathayil, "Deriving Morality from Politics: Rethinking the Formula of Humanity."

39. *Groundwork*, 4:429.

40. *Groundwork*, 4:403.

41. *Groundwork,* 4:429–30

42. I can provide a very rough account, though, about how this might go. To show that my acting in a way against which another person has a right necessarily uses them in some way, we would have to show that I *must* regard that person's rightful freedom as an extension of the person himself. I think it is possible to show this just in the case that I have already agreed to that person's domain of rightful freedom as something that is strictly inseparable from his status as a moral equal endowed with innate right. Kant can show this only after he has given the argument for the necessity of entering a civil condition. Once we have entered a civil condition, a person's actual rights, as laid down and made conclusive in a civil condition, are rights that I must agree to in order to fully respect the other's right to innate freedom. My assent to understanding his or her rights as an extension of his or her moral equality is explained by my assent to those rights through a united and general will, which is something I have a duty of right to consent to. Because I have agreed to these rights already through a united and general will, it creates a practical contradiction to say that I can act in a way inconsistent with those rights without understanding myself to have *used* him; I have already

consented to a system of rights in which affecting what is rightfully his is using his freedom itself, and not just doing something that merely affects him.

43. There are some familiar cases where consent can be tacit or assumed. As I understand it, consent is still necessary in these cases, but it is not obtained in the usual way, either because it is inconvenient or because it is impossible to obtain for some reason. For example, when I buy a magazine at the grocery store, I physically hand money to the clerk, who hands me the magazine, and I exit the store with the magazine, even though no one verbally agreed to the transaction. In such a case, consent is tacit: our actions demonstrate the existence of consent, without either party having to verbally give it. This is possible because we share an understanding of what it means to give consent in such a case. Consent is still strictly required: I cannot just walk out of the store without paying for the magazine and claim that the clerk didn't object and so must have consented, for example. The clerk gives tacit consent by accepting my payment, not by simply omitting complaint about me leaving with the magazine. In cases of assumed consent it is much the same: physicians assume consent to emergency treatment, for example, because most people want this, and it is often impossible to obtain actual consent. But in cases where there is reason to believe a person did not consent to such treatment (if there is a written DNR order, for example) then the assumption is overturned, and treatment is not justifiable.

44. *Groundwork*, 4:429–30.

45. This overlap should not be surprising. Kant seems to understand "perfect duties to others" as basically overlapping with the set of duties of right. We can see evidence of this, for example, in the way that the *Metaphysics of Morals* is organized. The second half, the *Doctrine of Virtue*, is divided into three basic sections: imperfect and perfect duties to self, and imperfect duties to others. Notably missing is a section on perfect duties to others, which is, implicitly, contained in the first half of the book—the *Doctrine of Right*.

46. In a civil condition, of course, there can be legitimate limits on the means by which I protect my property.

47. This may seem like an extreme example to some readers, but almost everyone thinks that such actions are justifiable in at least some cases. It may be necessary to shoot armed persons who wage war on me or invade my home hoping to harm me, for example. When the use of deadly force is justifiable is something that is in principle subject to determination by the united and general will through the political process. So, if it is illegal to shoot trespassers in a civil condition, then on this account shooting a trespasser would necessarily use them as a mere means; they have a right against this, as determined through the political process. However, there is no a priori argument against shooting trespassers in a state of nature, which is a good thing because if such behavior were categorically impermissible then Kant could not justify the use of lethal force in cases where a trespasser is likely to cause great harm, such as in the above examples, and otherwise could not be stopped.

48. My account here consequently differs from the argument given by Japa Pallikkathayil, who claims that "one treats another merely as a means if and only if one either (1) violates her rights [i.e., as determined by law] or (2) expresses the denial of the claim that the person has equal practical standing in virtue of her humanity." I

agree with (1), although for somewhat different reasons than Pallikkathayil gives. (2), however, is too restrictive. Pallikkathayil argues that expressing a denial of someone's "equal practical standing" occurs in three cases: arrogance, defamation, and ridicule. However, there is no reason to limit using someone as a mere means to these kinds of overt and public cases. The Formula of Humanity prohibits intentionally treating others in any way that is premised on them being mere means. Since there are myriad ways of acting that *could* be motivated by making others a mere means to our ends, just about any action could theoretically run afoul of the mere means clause. See Pallikkathayil, "Deriving Morality from Politics: Rethinking the Formula of Humanity."

49. Tom L. Beauchamp and James F. Childress, *Principles of Biomedical Ethics*, 7th ed. (New York: Oxford University Press, 2013), 138.

50. O'Neill, "Kant and the Social Contract Tradition."; Louis Philippe Hodgson, "Kant on the Right to Freedom: A Defense," *Ethics* 120, no. 4 (2010); Pallikkathayil, "Deriving Morality from Politics: Rethinking the Formula of Humanity."

Chapter 7

Kidney Markets and the Limits of Legitimacy

With accounts of political legitimacy and authority, we can now turn to practical and important questions about the laws and policies governing health care. In this chapter we will consider the legal permissibility of markets in kidneys, and in chapter 8, the laws governing informed consent in the clinical context.

For Kant the major questions respecting the legal permissibility of a market in kidneys revolve around the legitimacy of the government. In this chapter I will explore two limitations that Kant's theory of legitimacy imposes on governments, and the implications of these limitations for the legal permissibility of a kidney market. First, Kant's theory of legitimacy imposes limits on the government's right to prohibit the voluntary exchanges involving human kidneys. Because voluntary exchanges affect only the rights and freedoms of those engaging in the exchange, attempts to prohibit such exchanges are themselves contrary to right. Second, Kant's theory of legitimacy imposes limits on the government's ability to enforce contracts. While most contracts can be enforced because of the way in which they alter the rights and duties of the contracting parties, some contracts cannot be enforced because they would require persons to violate their own "internal duties of right." Contracts that promise the delivery of a living person's integral body parts, such as kidneys, violate internal duties of right. Because of these limitations issuing from the theory of legitimacy, the government can neither prohibit kidney sales nor enforce contracts for such sales.

To keep this chapter as simple as possible, I focus here on exchanges involving human kidneys. Human kidney sales represent the simplest kind of organ sales because kidney transplants need not substantially harm the kidney vendor. However, as I will discuss briefly at the end of this chapter, most of the considerations treated here likely apply to sales involving other organs as well.

CONSENT AND LEGITIMATE PROHIBITIONS

United Choice and Consent

In previous chapters, we have seen how Kant develops an account of persons' rights in a state of nature—persons can have rights to their persons and their property, because such rights can coexist with the freedom of everyone under universal law. Rights to persons and property also entail general rights to alter those rights, and so to alter what belongs to each—by giving gifts or making exchanges, for example. Changing our respective rights requires what Kant calls a "united choice." A united choice consists, first, in a choice. As we saw in chapter 5, Kant distinguishes a "choice" from a "mere wish."[1] A wish refers to my internal state of affairs, my desires or needs. I may *wish* to spend my paycheck on a trip to the Bahamas. But my *choice* is to spend most of my paycheck on rent. I exercise a choice when I set my means toward some end. It is presumably the fruit of (at least) some of my wishes, but there is no reason to inquire closely into the relationship between a person's choices and his or her wishes. Kant specifies that the concept of right is concerned with only the *form* of a choice (that is, whether it can formally coexist with the free actions of others) and not its *matter* (that is, the ends toward which the action is oriented).[2] Right is concerned with what I actually do, not with what I hope to achieve by it.

To be rightful, my choices affecting others' rights must be *united* with the choice of those whose rights they affect. This means, essentially, that others must agree, in unison with my choice, to alter their rights in the relevant way. That the choice be united is both a necessary and sufficient condition for ensuring the rightfulness of the choice.

It is necessary that the choice be united because if it were not, then the free choice of one person could not coexist with the freedom of the other and so would violate the Universal Principle of Right. So I cannot choose to buy a car from you, unless you also choose to sell it. Choosing to buy your car without your corresponding choice to sell it (to me, for the sum agreed upon) is theft. It does not matter whether I left what I considered a fair sum in your mailbox as compensation, or even if you would have accepted this offer. What matters is whether you actually did accept the offer.

The existence of a united choice is also sufficient for ensuring that the interaction is rightful. By characterizing a choice as "united," Kant indicates that all the parties whose rights are affected by the interaction make the choice together. The rights of third parties are, by definition, not directly affected by the interaction. Why is the united choice of all the parties whose rights are affected sufficient for ensuring rightfulness? *All* the duties of right are summarized by the Universal Principle of Right, namely, that each person must act externally in ways that can coexist with the freedom of others, in accordance with a universal law. Right is dichotomous in the sense that actions are either right or not right; there is no third category. Because actions that do not violate the Universal Principle of Right are fundamentally in accordance with right, Kant says that persons are "authorized to do to others anything that does not in itself diminish what is theirs."[3] The *only* relevant question, as far as right is concerned, is whether an action violates others' rights.

When united choice is present, then, it can justify interactions that would otherwise be non-rightful. In this way it plays a role similar to the one that consent plays in law. Consent, on Kant's account,[4] is important because it makes it possible for interactions between persons to remain essentially free, while simultaneously remaining compatible with the freedom of everyone.

To refer to "consent" in the context of bioethics is to invite references to the moral concept of autonomy. However, the Kantian account of legally relevant consent does not depend on its relationship to autonomy, and it is worth briefly discussing why. First, "consent" does not depend on the concept of autonomy as Kant describes it in his moral writings. For Kant, an autonomous choice is a choice in accordance with the moral law. But a rightful consent is not necessarily one that is given on the basis of maxims one can will as a universal law, nor need it be one that treats all involved persons as ends rather than mere means. I rightfully consent just if my choice is compatible with the (external) freedom of everyone, according to universal law.

Second, Kantian consent does not depend on the concept of autonomy as it is usually discussed and defended in bioethics. Prominent accounts of informed consent in bioethics have generally relied on accounts of autonomy other than Kant's. Beauchamp and Childress, for example, ground informed consent in a conception of nonideal autonomy, intended only to ensure that a person's choice is his or her own, rather than that of someone else.[5] On Beauchamp and Childress's account, someone's threat to fire, divorce, alienate, withhold some benefit, or visit any other unpleasant (but otherwise rightful) consequence on me might be thought to undermine autonomy, because such threats involve manipulation. Decisions I make following instances of manipulation by others are best characterized, perhaps, as not authentically mine. But for Kant, what matters is not ultimately the authenticity of my decision; rather, what matters is that I make the final choice, and that my final choice has not been conditioned by someone else's violation of my freedom under universal law. So threats to visit some unpleasant (but otherwise rightful) consequence on me if I do not comply with a request do not undermine the validity of my subsequent consent. Threats to visit me with consequences that are non-rightful (for example, a threat to maim or to steal), however, invalidate a subsequent consent.

Rights to Body Parts

Because united choice is both necessary and sufficient for rightfulness, persons may engage in consensual interactions—they may give, trade, buy, or sell that to which they have rights—so long as they find others who also consent to the interaction. This suggests, at least prima facie, that individuals have a right to sell organs such as kidneys.

This might be thought to raise a question, however, about whether persons have rights to their bodies in the relevant sense to allow such transactions. Many people will agree that we have rights to our bodies, in some sense. But it seems that we can distinguish between rights of noninterference and property rights, for example. Are human bodies—or pieces of them, like kidneys—things that belong to us, that we can sell by contract or exchange just as we exchange baseball cards or cross-country skis? As we saw in chapter 4, some of those commenting on Kant's view of organ sales have pointed out that Kant distinguished sharply between persons (as their bodies) and things, a distinction that is crucial to Kant's explanation of the special moral prohibitions against selling body parts. Couldn't Kant use this same distinction in his political philosophy to ground legal prohibitions against selling humans or their constitutive body parts?

The distinction between persons and things does retain an important place in Kant's political philosophy. In short, Kant's theory of right requires that we treat persons differently from things because persons are capable of free choice, and so we must not interfere with their external freedom. We do not have similar duties toward things which, by themselves, make no normative claims on us. Moreover, our rights to our own bodies are stronger than our rights to our property. The right I have to my body is a result of the fact that it is the extension of my person in time and space: I just am my body. For Kant, human bodies are special because of the kind of bodies they are. The normal adult human body has rational capacities, and because it has rational capacities it is subject to the moral law and has free choice. As I argued in chapter 6, it is because rationality is innate in human beings that they have an innate right to freedom. Kant distinguishes between the innate right we have to our persons and the acquired right we have in everything else.[6] The distinction is important because, as Kant puts it, in cases where an acquired right conflicts with someone's innate right, the burden of proof falls on the one who seems to be infringing on another's innate right.[7] Consequently, innate right should be understood to enjoy priority over acquired right.

However, as I discussed in chapter 5, both bodies and property are within the domain or sphere of a person's rightful freedom. This means that, from the outside, we have a duty to respect the freedom of others to do what they want with either their property or their bodies. To infringe on either would be to violate the rights of the right holder.

This similarity is not premised on the idea that people have the same kinds of interests in their bodies as they do in things. If Kantian rights depended on the importance or quality of interests that they protect, then we might be able to decide or discover what sort of interests people have in either bodies or things and then force them to use what is theirs to achieve these interests (or, alternatively, forcibly to prevent them from using their bodies or things in ways contrary to their interests). Kant does not deny that people have interests in bodies and things. But for Kant, the idea of a "right" means the right-holder has sole authority to decide what interest she will take in that which is rightfully hers. The ability to exercise this authority and to simultaneously exclude all others from making decisions with respect to a thing that is rightfully hers is the whole meaning of having a "right." And in this respect, bodies and objects are identical. If a right holder is not authorized to exclude others from a body which is rightfully her own, she does not really have a right to it. If another gets to tell her what ends she will pursue with her body, then the other has a right to it in a way that she does not. For a third party to say, then, that a person has a right to her body but not in the sense that would allow her to trade or sell it, would be to detract from her innate right, and, practically to assert partial ownership over her in her body.

Prohibiting Purchases

It could be objected that even if a person can sell an organ, this does not demonstrate anyone has a right to buy them. Perhaps the government cannot prohibit sales but can prohibit purchases. In some jurisdictions governments have done this for sex work: selling sexual services is not criminalized, but buying them is.

The objection is plausible, particularly because as we have just seen, Kant drew a systematic division between innate right, which includes a right to one's own body, and acquired right, which is our rights to things external to ourselves, such as property, contracts, and money. Kant also thought that acquired right is subject to the state's ratification. The state, acting as the embodiment of the united will, can conclusively settle who owns some piece of property or can determine that some property or good belongs to all in common. It is for this reason that possession of any piece of property is only "provisional" until what belongs to each is conclusively established in a civil condition.[8] Similarly, the state can decide when private resources become public resources through taxation.[9] So, it might be thought that if the state can go so far as to garnish some part of an individual's income through taxation, for example, then the state could also put limitations on how individuals use their income.

Although it is true that the state has authority to determine what is "laid down as right,"[10] it does so in a way that is meant to reaffirm or make conclusive what could be determined as right in a state of nature (according to the principles of right discussed in chapters 5 and 6). "Public right" is a system of laws that needs to be "promulgated" by the state to bring about a rightful condition.[11] Kant treats issues such as the police power, taxation, and welfare under this heading. These laws, however, do not result in any genuinely new powers for the state; rather, public right "contains no further or other duties of human beings among themselves than can be conceived in [private right]."[12] Consequently, powers that seem new (such as the power of taxation) are conceived of as subsidiary to the overall purpose of the state to preserve itself,[13] which is in turn necessary for securing the requirements of private right. Thus, although the state has the authority to determine that a portion of my income must be returned to the state for the purpose of preserving the state, it does not at any point acquire the authority to tell me what I may do with that which remains in my possession. Indeed, the only reason the state has the authority to tax in the first place is so that it can protect external freedom, that is, the freedom of individuals to use what is theirs according to their own plans and purposes. In sum, then, the state cannot prohibit purchases for the same reason it cannot prohibit sales: the state exists to protect persons' external freedom in both their bodies and their property. So long as organ sales do not infringe on the freedom of nonconsenting parties, the government lacks a legitimate basis for prohibiting them.

Kidney Sales and the Poor

Another potential objection is that legally permitting kidney sales would result in a market characterized by poor sellers and wealthy buyers. Since Kant thinks that the state has a duty to protect those are unable to "maintain" themselves, his view could permit prohibitions on kidney sales for the purpose of protecting the most vulnerable members of society.

To respond to this worry, we should briefly review what Kant says about welfare rights. It is important to note that Kant does not divide persons up into "poor" and "rich," but instead distinguishes between the class of persons who are not able to meet their own "most necessary natural needs" and everyone else.[14] Those unable to meet their own needs have a right to sustenance from the state, because persons could not agree to a a civil condition in which it would be possible for them to become so disenfranchised that they could not meet their own needs. Someone who cannot meet his or her own needs would be more independent in a state of nature, where exclusion from the property of others is circumstantial, inconsistent, and disputed, rather than the result of a thoroughgoing social coordination. Others have a corresponding duty to meet the needs of those who cannot meet their own, because the civil condition, by protecting property and other rights, plays a role in maintaining their wealth much as it does in maintaining the needs of these persons. So some welfare rights are necessary within a civil condition, because no one can have a duty to submit to a civil condition in which they are entirely dependent on others for exercising even their most basic freedoms, and no one has a right to wealth if it makes others dependent in this way.[15]

If persons are unable to maintain themselves, then, the Kantian prescription is that the state should meet their basic needs. Prohibiting organ sales would be an extremely indirect way of meeting their needs—indeed, it isn't clear how it would help meet them at all—but it would also be ultimately unnecessary, since their needs must be met in other ways.

But what about those who are relatively poor but whose basic needs have been met? Two kinds of concerns might be raised about sales made by those persons. First, we might worry that their organ sales will be unfree, that is, essentially coerced in some way. In other words, we might worry that sales by these persons will not reflect their true or authentic preferences, in a way that would not concern us if they were better off. However, on Kant's view, a person's freedom is measured not by the amount of money they have in comparison to others, but instead by the freedom they have to exercise sovereignty over what is in their domain, free of the interfering decisions of others. This freedom is external freedom, or freedom from others. Persons whose basic needs are met and whose rights are protected by the rule of law within a civil condition are capable of living independently of others, even when they have less than average. If it were true that being relatively poor invalidated the authenticity and so rightfulness of a person's decisions, this would be a problem not only for selling organs, but for any decisions made by such a person at all. However, on Kant's view the poor are just as entitled to freedom as the rich are, and this means that they have just as much right as anyone to sell their organs. If anyone is entitled to sell their organs, then everyone is.

On the other hand, the concern might be instead that no one has a right to sell organs, but that it is only the poor who will do so. This would beg the question, since what is in question is whether there is a right to sell organs. If there is no right to sell organs, then the question is: why not? Two possible answers seem evident: either because such sales are morally wrong, or because it is not in anyone's true interest to sell organs. As we have already seen, the fact that sales are morally wrong is no reason to legally prohibit them. The Categorical Imperative cannot be enforced because it is not possible to coerce someone to act for duty's sake (see chapter 4). As far as interests go, we have already seen that people have rights only to their external freedom. External freedom is freedom from others' determinations about what is in our interests. So, persons actually have rights to be free of paternalistic determinations about whether it is in their interests to sell their organs. Paternalistic laws are one of the few things that Kant himself categorically rejects as incompatible with rights.[16]

Exchanges for Body Parts

If persons have a broad right to exercise their united choice with consenting others to alter their respective relationships toward anything to which they currently have rights, and if persons have rights to their bodies and their finances, to use them and dispose of them in accordance with their own purposes, then persons have a right to sell and buy body parts.

Consequently, on the Kantian view, laws prohibiting the sale of organs—present in nearly all developed nations—must be understood to violate persons' rights. For example, in the United States, 42 US Code § 274e provides that "it shall be unlawful for any person to knowingly acquire, receive, or otherwise transfer any human organ for valuable consideration for use in human transplantation." Here the law prohibits private parties from selling body parts to others. However, contrary to the way in which Kant has been understood by the vast majority of commentators, not only does Kant's philosophy not support these legal prohibitions, it also shows why they are impossible. Prohibiting such exchanges violates the right of the exchangers because it infringes on free choices that can coexist with the freedom of everyone under universal laws.

In fact, the point could be put even more strongly. Innate right is itself the font of state authority. As described in chapters 5 and 6, it is only because persons have an innate right to coercively resist those who would interfere in their freedom that it is permissible for states to coerce at all. States accrue the authority to coerce by virtue of their representing the citizens who collectively have the authority to join together under a system of universal rights. A state that forcibly prohibits persons from using what is theirs for their own purposes corrodes the very foundation of its own authority: the protection of a system of equal freedom according to universal laws for all. Such a state actively asserts that it possesses its citizens. It tells them the ends that they must pursue with their persons, and thus, exercises partial ownership over them in their persons.

CONTRACTS AND LEGITIMATE ENFORCEMENT

On Kant's account of the legitimate purposes of the state, then, persons must be legally permitted to determine the ends for which their bodies and belongings may be used. Moreover, they have broad authority to authorize others to use what belongs to them and may even go so far as to transfer body parts to others in consensual exchanges.

However, insofar as persons exchange something of value for something else of value, their conduct is usually understood as a kind of *contract*. Because contracts alter the legal rights and obligations of the individuals who are party to them, courts enforce them. If two parties enter into a contract and one party breaches the contract, then the party who breaches the contract is forced to compensate the other party for the breach.

Enforcing contracts seems problematic, however, where those contracts involve the sale of human body parts. For example, consider a case where a contracting buyer's life depends on receiving a kidney itself (and not just the economic benefit attached to the kidney). If the vendor changes his or her mind about selling it at the last minute, courts might be forced to consider an order for specific performance—that is, ordering forcible removal and delivery of the kidney—which, not unlike a legal demand for a "pound of flesh,"[17] is an altogether ugly prospect. But even requiring compensation for breach of contract in such cases seems problematic. As we saw in chapter 3, on Kant's view persons have a perfect moral duty toward themselves not to sell parts of their body. A state that forced persons to compensate buyers for breached contracts involving kidneys would be in the awkward position of forcing persons to compensate others for a failure to do something that is deeply immoral, which doesn't seem much better than forcing them to do the immoral thing in the first place. While Kant's political philosophy allows that many actions can be right without necessarily being morally good, it would seem problematic if one of the implications of his political theory was that persons can enlist the state's assistance to force others to do things that are necessarily immoral or to pay for a failure to do them.

Kant's political philosophy provides the resources to explain why consensual transactions for kidneys are permissible while also addressing some of the problems that might be thought to accompany such consensual transactions, such as the enforcement of contracts for kidney sales. Much like his view on the rightfulness of kidney sale prohibitions, Kant's view about the possibility of enforcing such contracts is a consequence of his view of the limits of government legitimacy. For Kant, even though contracts for body parts cannot be prevented, they also cannot be enforced. To see why they cannot be enforced, we shall look first at Kant's general explanation of the structure of contracts, and then show why internal duties of right prevent the enforcement of contracts for human body parts.

Consent and Contracts

Contracts, for Kant, are the general means by which one person acquires something from someone else.[18] Contracts can exist in right because they involve the "united choice" of both of those whose rights are affected. In this sense, they are a species of consent.[19]

One of the distinguishing features of contracts is that they constitute agreements about a future alteration of our respective rights. The change in our rights may happen immediately after conclusion of the contract, but often it does not. Accordingly, Kant describes a contract as consisting first in a *promise*. The promise puts each party under an obligation for the performance of some action in the future. This could be a promise to do a set amount of work, to render payment for a certain amount of work, to deliver some object into the other's possession, or whatever. However, the promise does not itself create a right to the thing promised.[20] Instead, performance of the action promised is necessary before the thing (whether funds, labor, an object, a title, and so on) is actually transferred into the possession of the other and becomes his by right. Kant calls this performance *delivery*.[21]

The two major parts to a contract, promise and delivery, have distinct implications for right. Subsequent to the promise but before the delivery, I possess only a right against a specific person, for a future performance: it is a right to the other's "freedom and means."[22] It is not until the performance or "delivery" occurs that I obtain a right to the thing, namely, a right against *everyone* with respect to the object transferred into my possession.

In many contracts the two parts are not obviously distinct because the promise and delivery happen nearly simultaneously. When I buy a book at the bookstore, for example, the book is already in my physical possession when I walk up to the counter. After paying for it, it is mine. The stages to the contract—the promise and subsequent delivery—happen simultaneously, and in most cases, seamlessly.

The distinction between promise and delivery is more significant in cases where the promise and the delivery are separated by more time. For example, it may be that I have ordered from you a book of which you have several copies. However, it need not be the case that I have bought any particular copy of the book. Rather, what I have bought is a right against you to the delivery of a copy of the book into my possession. You could even sell all of your inventory, and consequently have no copy left of the book that I bought, but as long as you obtain another copy somewhere and deliver it to me by the time promised, you have fulfilled the contract.

On the other hand, perhaps you have bought something specific from me. Kant uses the example of a horse: perhaps you have purchased a specific horse from me, to be delivered some time in the future. If the horse dies or becomes sick before the delivery, the seller bears the risk.[23] If, on the other hand, our contract has arranged for me to pick it up at such and such a time, and I fail to show up, then at that time the seller may regard me as the rightful owner of the horse and the bearer of risk associated with it. Similarly, if fire, theft, or something else destroys the thing you have promised to me; or, if you yourself cannot acquire the thing you promised because someone else breaches their contract with you, none of these by themselves relieve you of your obligation to me. The thing promised remains your responsibility until you have delivered it safely to me, in the manner we have agreed on.

Persons have rights to make binding promises for the same general reasons that they have rights to consent to the use of things that belong to them by right. In the same way that persons have present rights to their bodies and possessions, persons have rights to their future selves and means as well, and thus can consent to use of these in a "promise." When two persons make a united choice concerning their respective future performances, they promise to each other things to which they each have respective rights. Because their united choice concerns only that to which each has respective rights, and this choice does not interfere with the rights of others, their contract is compatible with the freedom of everyone.

Because each party to a contract conditions her promises on the promise of the other—each party must offer, in contemporary terms, "consideration," that is, something in exchange—failure by one party to deliver what was promised means that the choice is no longer "united." Of course, normally a failure to unite in a choice just means that there is no contract and so no alteration of rights. Since the actual delivery of the promise has not occurred yet, it may seem like persons could just unilaterally dissolve contracts. However, as we have already seen, after the promise but before the delivery there has been an actual change in rights, despite the fact that there is no change yet in property: each party acquires a right against the "freedom and means" of the other party. So, although the contract I form when I order a book does not yet entitle me to any particular book, I *do* currently have a right against you that your current (and continuing) use of whatever freedom and means you have be consistent with your ability to deliver the promised book to me. Similarly, I have a duty to use my freedom and means in a way that is consistent with delivering payment to you. If I constrain my use of my freedom and means in order to fulfill my duty toward you, but I do not receive what I am owed in the contract, *which was the condition for my constraining my means in the first place,* then you have wronged me. Your failure to perform is not compatible with my freedom. As a result, I have the subsequent right either to force you to perform the sale or to compensate me for the breached promise.

Keeping promises in contracts is thus not legally obligatory as a result of the moral obligation to keep promises, as some "Kantian" accounts of contracts would have it.[24] Nor are they obligatory because of societally defined moral responsibilities associated with receiving some benefit.[25] Contracts, as a species of consent, are rightful interactions insofar as they involve a united choice. Keeping contracts is obligatory because persons have the authority to contract with others to alter their legal obligations and rights. And the promisee in a contract has a right to enforce the contract because, by failing to fulfill his end of the bargain, the breaching promisor has essentially made the promisee's freedom subject to his own.

If a kidney vendor could form contracts for the sale of organs in the same way he forms contracts for other things, then, by his promise he would create an obligation against his own freedom and means, in this case to dismember himself and deliver the promised organ. The promisee would simultaneously gain a right to the performance of the dismemberment and subsequent delivery of the organ. However, because persons' bodies are integrally related to their ability to hold rights and duties at all, such contracts pose special problems for a theory of right or justice. On Kant's view, although such sales can't be prohibited, they nevertheless violate what he calls *internal duties of right*. The existence of such internal duties explains why the government's authority cannot extend to the enforcement of contracts for a person's kidney or other integral body parts.

Limits on the Enforcement of Contracts

Internal Duties of Right

The Universal Principle of Right seems to suggest that persons have no legal duties except to restrain their actions when these conflict with the freedom of others. There is, however, an exception to this rule. Persons have internal duties of right,[26] which forbid them from doing anything incompatible with their own status as a right holder.

It seems that such duties must be a necessary corollary to innate right. In chapter 6 I discussed innate right as the foundation for other rights. It is only because persons have a right to be free of others in general, that they can have rights to be free of others in specific ways. We have duties corresponding to the innate right in others, then, not only not to interfere with the specific rights that people have, but to treat them generally as persons capable of having legal rights and duties.

Since the individual himself is one of these people who have this duty, there is a reflexive duty, or a duty toward himself, to treat himself as a right holder. Consequently, the individual has a duty toward himself to refrain from doing anything that treats himself as less than a legal person, that is, as a thing that is not capable of holding rights. In other words, he has duties to refrain from doing any of the multiple things that might derogate his status as a right holder.

What sorts of actions might an individual commit that would suggest he or she is less than a full right holder? Kant does not give a systematic overview of these in the *Doctrine of Right*, but his view can nevertheless be pieced together from his comments.

First, we should notice that Kant uses the phrase "internal duties" to denote the class of duties associated with being an "honorable human being."[27] Whichever of these terms is preferred,[28] Kant comments that this class of duties is just the "obligation from the right of humanity in our own person."[29] This identification is important, because Kant elsewhere also associates "perfect [moral] duties to oneself" as following from the right of humanity in our own person.[30] If internal duties of right follow from the right of humanity in our own person, and so do perfect duties to oneself, then it seems likely that the formal duties contained in these two groups (internal duties of right and perfect duties to oneself) are roughly the same.

Let us suppose that this reading of Kant is correct. It is still a surprising finding: why would internal duties of right contain the same formal duties as perfect duties to oneself? In addition to the textual reasons for thinking these groups contain the same formal duties, we can give a philosophical reason, too.

Both sets of duties emerge from what it means to Kant to be a person. A person, for Kant, is someone whose actions can be imputed to him; this definition of person is common to both his moral and political philosophy.[31] In other words, a person is a causality, the origin of free actions.[32]

In the legal context, this means that a person can be understood as the source of legally relevant actions: a person can make legal claims on others, and others can make legal claims on her. The person is someone who can thus own property, enter contractual or otherwise consensual relationships with others, and so on. A person is someone with the status of a right holder, in other words. Persons are thus sharply distinguished from things: things cannot be the source of legally relevant actions. They cannot hold rights and cannot be the sources of legal claims made on persons, nor the recipients of such legal claims. Internal duties of right are those duties persons have toward themselves that follow from their status as legal persons, or their innate right. They require that persons refrain from actions that necessarily treat themselves as mere things, that is, as less than legal persons, or right holders.

In the moral context, similarly, a person is the source of morally relevant actions. Such a person is subject to moral duties, and also possessed of moral rights against others. Perfect duties to oneself are those moral duties persons have toward themselves that follow from this status as a moral person. They require that persons refrain from actions that necessarily treat themselves as mere things, that is, as less than moral persons, or ends in themselves.

Because Kant understands certain kinds of actions necessarily to treat persons as things (rightly or wrongly; as we discussed in chapter 3, many have questioned whether Kant commits the fallacy of division when inferring obligations not to sell body parts from an obligation not to sell the whole body), committing one of these actions will violate *both* internal duties of right and perfect duties to oneself at the same time. So, it should not be surprising that the two groups of duties overlap in the formal duties they require. Both sets of duties emerge quite naturally from the fundamental distinction between persons and things, which is a distinction relevant to both Kant's moral and political philosophy. They both require, basically, not doing anything that *necessarily* treats a person as a mere thing.

What kinds of actions necessarily treat persons as things? For Kant there is a long list of such items.[33] Most importantly for the present topic, self-mutilation, or partial suicide—and so, as we have seen, *organ sales and donations*—treat persons as mere things. Subsequently, kidney sales and donations violate not only perfect duties to oneself, but also internal duties of right. They treat persons as mere things, and so, less than ends in themselves (when considered in the moral context) and less than full right holders (when considered in the legal context).

It is important to bear in mind, however, that because the two classes of duties are regarded from different viewpoints, they are distinct in some ways. Internal duties of right are legal obligations, and perfect duties to oneself are moral obligations. These are different kinds of obligations, as we saw in chapter 4. Furthermore, by describing perfect duties to oneself only in the *Doctrine of Virtue* and not the *Doctrine of Right*, Kant makes clear that he thinks these moral duties "cannot be enforced."[34] Right has only to do with the practical relation between persons,[35] and so does not forbid self-regarding actions, even when these violate internal duties of right. Consequently, although persons have internal duties of right to refrain from selling organs, because internal duties of right are owed only to oneself, they cannot ultimately be enforced.

Impossible Obligations

If internal duties of right cannot be enforced, then why do they appear at all in Kant's political philosophy? They occur here because although they cannot be directly enforced, they nevertheless have implications for legal relationships between people. Most pertinent to the topic at hand, internal duties of right have implications for the kinds of contracts that can be enforced. Specifically, the existence of these duties makes it impossible for individuals to create contractual obligations that conflict with them.

Imagine a contract in which one party sells a kidney to another. Such a sale is immoral for Kant because it violates perfect duties to oneself, insofar as it constitutes "partially murdering oneself," and so "debas[es] humanity in one's person."[36] On the argument I have given, such a sale presumably also violates an internal duty of right insofar as it treats a person as a thing that can be bought and sold, rather than as a legal subject and right holder.

Because a promise normally creates an obligation on the part of the promisor to deliver something, a promise to sell a kidney would, theoretically, create an obligation for the promisor to cut out a part of her body and deliver it to the buyer. However, because she promises something that she has a preexisting obligation (due to an internal duty of right) not to do, by promising to deliver the kidney the promisor creates an obligation to do something that she also has an obligation not to do. If it were possible to create such an obligation, then a person would have an obligation to both do and not do the same thing.

Conflicting duties of right are problematic because they necessarily rely on conflicting rights. So, my internal duty not to divide my body comes from my innate right, my right as a unified, whole body not to have anything done to it which implies that it is less than a unified right-holder. My duty to cut out part of my body comes from your right to that which was promised you in our contract. Your right to have my kidney delivered to you conflicts with my right not to have my kidney cut out by anyone, including me. If I have a right not to do something, it cannot also be the case that you have a right to my doing that exact same thing. Such a promise is impossible, then, because I do not have the authority to create a duty that conflicts with my own innate right.

Because it is impossible for me to create such an obligation, a promisee cannot even demand compensation for breach of contract in the case that the promisor fails to deliver a kidney. Breach of contract assumes that a person had an obligation to fulfill what was promised in the contract but failed to do so. But if a person does not have the authority to create such an obligation, because he is not authorized to relinquish his internal duties of right, then he did not succeed in creating such an obligation, and he cannot be forced to compensate anyone for failing to deliver what was promised. Moreover, if it is impossible to create an obligation to deliver a promised kidney, then enforcement of such a putative obligation would force someone to do something they have no obligation to do. In this way, it would also violate that person's innate right.

Kant considers the possibility of enforcing contracts that violate our internal duties of right (or "the right of humanity in our own person") in a passage that considers contracts for concubinage and prostitution:

> neither concubinage nor hiring a person for enjoyment on one occasion . . . is a contract that could hold in right. As for the latter, everyone will admit that a person who has concluded such a contract could not rightfully be held to the fulfillment of her promise if she regrets it. So with regard to the former, a contract to be a concubine . . . also comes to nothing . . . Accordingly, either party can cancel the contract with the other as soon as it pleases without the other having grounds for complaining about any infringement of its rights.[37]

Although Kant considers here a contract which objectifies some or both parties (which is to say, it violates the "right of humanity in our own person," as Kant makes clear earlier in the same passage[38]), he does not conclude that this means that the relationship should be criminalized or otherwise prohibited. Nor does he argue that the contracts are null and void, in the sense that they would fail to demonstrate consent. Instead, he comments merely that the contract cannot be enforced and either party can "cancel" it.

Kant's approach to contracts for prostitution and concubinage reflects, I suggest, the Kantian approach to contracts in general that violate internal duties of right.[39] Such contracts can serve as a sign of consent, and thus, can excuse such exchanges from charges of criminal liability. However, the contract is not void in the contemporary legal sense, which would mean essentially that the contract is of no legal effect whatsoever, such as when a minor or other legally incompetent person "contracts" for something. The contract does have a legal effect, insofar as it registers the consent of the parties to the transaction. As argued in the first half of this chapter, the parties have a right to make such exchanges because of their general rights over their persons and property and their subsequent capacity to engage in interactions characterized by a united choice. The delivery of those things promised in the contract completes the transaction and provides further evidence that the exchange is a consensual one. However, the contract is unenforceable because the promise fails to create a legal duty. Individuals would, subsequently, be wrong to enforce such a contract, and so also cannot enlist the help of others or the state in enforcing such contracts.

Bodies and the Definition of Legal Persons

Contracts that necessarily objectify persons cannot be enforced, then, because it is impossible to create the duties on which enforcement would depend. The enforcement of such contracts would require that persons have the authority to create obligations to objectify themselves. But this they cannot do, because objectification violates one's own internal duties of right.

Although it may seem plausible to say in the abstract that any action that necessarily objectifies a legal person or subject could not form the basis of an enforceable contract, it may be doubted that kidney sales necessarily objectify persons. Kant undoubtedly thought that they do; but then again, Kant had a laundry list of actions that necessarily objectify persons, which included everything from prostitution and masturbation to selling one's hair. What are the reasons for thinking that selling a part of the human body—particularly a non-vital part, such as a redundant kidney—objectifies a person? The difficulties with any particular account of what a person is—and which body parts are essential to a person and so must never be treated as mere objects—will mount quickly, especially in an age where bodies are increasingly intertwined with a variety of devices, tissues, and transplanted organs.

As we saw in chapter 3, the question about the metaphysical status of different body parts is a philosophically controversial subject. I do not propose to resolve the debate here. Instead, I will merely point out that it is most plausible—at least, on a Kantian *political* account—that determining what constitutes a legal person, and what sorts of things objectify a legal person, will require an authoritative determination by the united and general will, through the political process.[40] In other words, what we require is a political decision, rather than a metaphysical or scientific discovery, about what constitutes a legal person. And so, we cannot claim in an a priori way—contrary to Kant's own implicit assumption, it seems—that kidneys or other body parts are part of a true legal self, rather than property or things attached to our bodies.

Is it reasonable to think that the united will would designate kidneys as *constituting* a legal person, rather than belonging (like property) to them? I think so. Kidneys are considered a part of a person in common law. Touching a person's property without consent is a trespass to chattel; touching a person's kidney or other body part without consent is battery. It seems that in both law and popular opinion, kidneys are usually understood as an integral part of legal subjects rather than mere objects attached to them. Actions that objectify embodied kidneys will presumably objectify persons as such. The conclusions I draw here about markets in kidneys, then, are plausible given what I take to be widely shared views of kidneys, but I note that this view of kidneys is subject to revision through political processes.

Consent: No Defense to Kidney Removal?

If this account of the internal duties of right is correct, then on a Kantian account kidney sales cannot be prohibited, but contracts for such sales should be considered unenforceable.

One commentator reaches a somewhat different conclusion about the implications of internal duties of right (or, as he calls them, "duties of rightful honor"[41]), however. Similar in some ways to the account I have offered, Ripstein's Kantian account holds that purely self-regarding actions, such as suicide, must be legally permitted, and he further holds that consent is a general justification for the rightfulness of legal interactions, according to the principle *volenti non fit iniuria*,[42] even when these interactions are usually considered harmful or otherwise inadvisable. If suicide and other self-regarding actions are legally permitted, and consent can justify interactions between legal persons, then one might think that voluntary euthanasia and virtually any other kind of consensual relationship, such as kidney sales, would have to be legal as well.

However, Ripstein argues that Kant's internal duties of right justify several exceptions to the general *volenti* rule. According to Ripstein, internal duties of right forbid the destruction of a person's own body, or as Ripstein calls it, a person's "purposiveness," because a person's purposiveness is the basis of a person's ability to form and implement any other purposes at all.[43] While suicide and other self-regarding actions (like, perhaps, self-removal of an organ) destroy a person's purposiveness and so violate internal duties of right, these actions are not the targets of public laws, according to Ripstein, because right has nothing to say about interactions with oneself, only interactions with others.[44] However, interactions *between* parties that require destroying the "purposiveness" of one or the other party are "normatively impossible." So, says Ripstein, on a Kantian account it turns out that consent is no defense to murder, slavery, or deliberate wounding or mutilation—these are "material exceptions" to the general rule permitting all consensual interactions.

Two important implications would seem to follow from Ripstein's view, if correct. First, Ripstein's view essentially justifies legal *prohibitions* against voluntary euthanasia, self-enslavement, and consensual wounding and mutilation: to say that "consent is no defense" is just to say that even when consent is present, these actions are still prohibited under the more general criminal laws that prohibit these actions when consent is *not* present. Second—although Ripstein does not consider it explicitly—it seems likely that, if consent is no defense to wounding or mutilation, then consent will also not be a defense to kidney donations or sales. Ripstein does think that some body-altering surgeries and permanent cosmetic procedures can be legally permitted.[45] But according to Ripstein, the legal permissibility of any particular body-altering procedure will depend on a political determination about whether it destroys part of an individual's "purposiveness," as a maiming would, or whether it is a harmless or even beneficial surgery, such as an ear piercing or appendectomy. Since surgeries necessary for retrieving kidneys are usually not intended to be of direct benefit to the organ donor/vendor, and put the donor/vendor at some degree of risk; and because kidneys are integral organs playing an important function, even if redundant; kidney removal for purposes of sale or donation are most naturally understood as mutilations that destroy an individual's purposiveness, and thus qualify as exceptions to the *volenti* rule and should (or at least, could) be legally prohibited on this view.

There are at least two serious problems with Ripstein's use of internal duties of right to justify prohibitions against any of the supposedly "material exceptions" to the volenti rule. The first problem is that Ripstein's conclusion about the legal prohibition of murder and slavery reaches significantly beyond his arguments. So Ripstein considers contracts and provides many good reasons why contracts that violate internal duties of right should not be enforced. Such contracts should not be enforced because, in Ripstein's terms, they contain "inconsistent terms" insofar as they treat persons as both legal right holders and mere objects.[46] While this treatment is perfectly satisfactory as a response to the enforcement of contracts, as I have also argued, it is unclear why Ripstein extends his conclusions further to allow for the prohibition and even legal punishment of transactions that were clearly consensual. It is one thing to say that a person cannot be held to a contract that requires his death; it is another to say that a person who kills with consent should be punished for murder.

Ripstein seemingly provides no argument for the latter claim. He suggests at one point that the reason such transactions cannot be allowed is that agents do not have the "normative power" to give consent to transactions requiring the violation of their internal duties of right.[47] If all Ripstein means by this is that such transactions violate internal duties of right, he is correct; the transaction is, in a sense, wrongful. But showing that the transaction is, in a sense, wrongful is not enough to show that the parties to the transaction should be subject to either coercive compensation or retribution by the state.

The question to be answered, to justify coercion, is this: Given the fact that the person wrongfully consented, does that person who wrongfully consented retain a right to coercively recover (either actually recover, or gain compensation for) whatever it is that he or she voluntarily gave away? (Showing that an individual does have this right is necessary for demonstrating the state's authorization to do the same, since the state's authorization to coerce proceeds from the individual's, as discussed in chapters 5 and 6.)

Ripstein's position implicitly assumes that the answer to this question is "yes," but it is by no means clear that is the correct one. A more plausible interpretation of the transaction is that the person who sold the organ (or consented to euthanasia, for example), by consenting to the transaction, implicitly waived any right to subsequent coercion of the other party.[48] If a person, by consenting, waives a right to future coercion, there remains no reason for the state to engage in coercive actions aimed at restoring the individual's rights either.

The second problem with Ripstein's account owes to the implausible implications of prohibiting actions that violate internal duties of right. Ripstein suggests that transactions that destroy the "purposiveness" of one actor or another can be prohibited because they violate internal duties of right. But internal duties of right, as we have seen, prohibit not just actions that destroy person's bodies, but any actions that necessarily fail to treat persons as full legal persons. For Kant, there is a huge list of such actions. If Ripstein were correct that all transactions involving these actions can be prohibited, this would mean that Kant thought that laws can prohibit, not only those transactions destroying a person's "purposiveness," but also all consensual transactions involving drunkenness, masturbation, and a host of other items that violate internal duties of right. But Kant never suggests this, and it seems unlikely that Kant held this position. The example shows that Ripstein's position, whatever its merits, has no clear basis in Kant, and so probably cannot serve to defend the "material exceptions" to the *volenti* rule in the way that Ripstein suggests. It should furthermore be noted that even if it turned out that Kant would have legally prohibited all transactions involving the violation of internal duties of right, then Ripstein would owe us an explanation about why he focuses only on violations that destroy purposiveness, and not all those that treat persons as less than full legal persons.

ENVISIONING A MARKET CHARACTERIZED BY UNENFORCEABLE CONTRACTS

Although one cannot create binding promises for one's kidney, the consensual delivery of kidneys cannot be prohibited. Once kidneys or other organs have been detached from the body of a legal person, they can no longer be considered parts of right-holding persons, and instead become things.[49] Once delivery of the organ occurs, it may even become the property of another person or, if transplanted into the body of another person, become a part of that person. Although the parties to the exchange may have written a contract prior to the transplant, no new rights or duties were created until the actual delivery of the kidney. Any written contract may serve as a testament that the organ vendor gave consent for the surgery that removed the kidney—albeit consent that she was entitled to revoke at any time prior to the actual operation as a consequence of her innate right. After the delivery, the transplant recipient presumably enjoys rights to the organ in the same way she enjoys rights to other parts of her body.

Non-enforceable contracts have been proposed before as a way of dealing with the difficulties involved in other contracts involving human bodies, such as contract motherhood or surrogacy.[50] The approach is also common in adoption law. If the Kantian account presented in this chapter is right, then it seems possible that market exchanges for not only surrogate wombs and adopted children but also kidneys and perhaps other sorts of body parts and personal services will have to be tolerated, even if such contracts treat persons as things and thus cannot be enforced. In any case, they could not be prevented merely on the grounds that they objectify persons and so violate the Categorical Imperative.

MORALITY, LEGITIMACY, AND BIOETHICS

Kant's remarks about the morality of organ donating and selling have long been the subject of vigorous debate in bioethics, in part because of the presumed implications of Kant's moral thought for policy and law. That so much effort has been expended in discovering the implications of Kant's moral philosophy for laws governing markets in kidneys is ironic, since as argued, Kant himself did not think that his moral philosophy had such implications, or that such a method of reasoning is the appropriate method for justifying policies or laws.

But more important than what position Kant would have ultimately taken is what Kant shows us about the relevance of political philosophy to questions about laws governing kidney transfers. For Kant, questions about laws and policies governing kidney distributions are first and foremost about whether the state can legitimately prevent persons from using their bodies in particular ways and whether it can enforce the relevant agreements between them. The conclusion which I have argued to be most consistent with Kant's view (that is, that limits on the state's authority require the legalization of kidney sales, but also, that contracts for such sales remain unenforceable) is poignant for illustrating the general point about the relevance of political philosophy. While readers may find the policy indicated by a Kantian analysis to be undesirable in some way or other, the fact that Kant reaches such seemingly disparate conclusions about what morality and rights require suggests that bioethics routinely overlooks foundational questions about the relationship between morality and the law. Kant demonstrates that reconceiving debates about the legal permissibility of kidney sales in terms of basic normative principles describing the nature and limits of government legitimacy—in other words, supplying some political philosophy—is the only way to give a full account of the stance laws should take toward kidney or other organ sales.

NOTES

1. 6:230.
2. 6:230.
3. 6:238.
4. Kant does not discuss a category of "consent," per se, although he frequently uses the term. I follow Ripstein here in using the term "consent" to refer to the broad category of interactions characterized by "united choice." Arthur Ripstein, *Force and Freedom: Kant's Legal and Political Philosophy* (Cambridge, Mass.: Harvard University Press, 2009), 111 ff.
5. Tom L. Beauchamp and James F. Childress, *Principles of Biomedical Ethics*, 7th ed. (New York: Oxford Univ. Press, 2013), 104–5 and 21 ff.
6. Kant implies that physically touching someone interferes with innate right at 6:248, which suggests that innate right includes a right to one's body.
7. 6:238.
8. 6:264–66.
9. 6:326.
10. 6:306.
11. 6:311.
12. 6:306.
13. 6:326.
14. 6:326.
15. This is one way of interpreting Kant's brief and cryptic remarks about why the state has a duty to maintain those who cannot meet their own needs. For other accounts and discussion, see Mary Gregor, "Kant on Welfare Legislation," *Logos* 6 (1985); Alexander Kaufman, *Welfare in the Kantian State* (New York: Oxford University Press, 1999); Ripstein, *Force and Freedom: Kant's Legal and Political Philosophy*, Ch. 9; Luke J Davies, "Kant on Welfare: Five Unsuccessful Defences," *Kantian Review* 25, no. 1 (2020). Although the reasons for and extent of welfare rights in the Kantian state are disputed, all that we need to know to respond to the current objection is that Kant thought that his view required meeting basic needs.
16. 6:317.
17. The difficulty in enforcing such a contract was one of the central plot elements in Shakespeare's *The Merchant of Venice*.
18. 6:271.
19. Ripstein, *Force and Freedom: Kant's Legal and Political Philosophy*, 111.
20. 6:274.
21. 6:274.
22. 6:274.
23. 6:275–76.
24. Charles Fried, *Contract as Promise: A Theory of Contractual Obligation* (Cambridge, Mass.: Harvard University Press, 1981), 16–17.
25. See Patrick S. Atiyah, *Promises, Morals, and Law* (New York: Oxford University Press, 1981).
26. 6:237.

27. See Kant's comment following the table outlining Ulpian's division of right, in which he characterizes Ulpian's three divisions as "internal duties, external duties, and duties that involve the derivation of the latter from the principle of the former by subsumption." 6:237. This comment identifies Ulpian's first imperative, to "be an honorable being," with what Kant calls "internal duties."

28. Ripstein, following Ulpian's phrase, uses the term "duties of rightful honor" instead of "internal duties of right" (*Force and Freedom: Kant's Legal and Political Philosophy*, Ch. 2, 136.) I prefer the term "internal duties" of right because it is the term Kant applies to these duties when he is not quoting Ulpian.

29. 6:237.

30. Perfect duties to oneself are indicated to correspond to the right of humanity in our own person in the table on 6:240.

31. Kant's definition is found in the introduction to the whole *Metaphysics of Morals*, not the introduction specific to the *Doctrine of Right*. 6:223.

32. For helpful discussion, see Jennifer K. Uleman, "External Freedom in Kant's "Rechtslehre": Political, Metaphysical," *Philosophy and Phenomenological Research* 68, no. 3 (2004).

33. In the *Doctrine of Virtue*, Kant mentions several vices including "murdering" oneself, the "unnatural use" of "sexual inclination," "excessive consumption of food and drink," and "lying, avarice, and false humility" (6:420). He discusses each of these vices in the following sections as those that "perfect duties to oneself" prohibit.

34. The *Doctrine of Virtue* contains those duties that cannot be the subject of an external lawgiving. See 6:219, *Doctrine of Virtue* 6:394. See also B. Sharon Byrd and Joachim Hruschka, *Kant's Doctrine of Right: A Commentary* (New York: Cambridge University Press, 2010), 63.

35. 6:230.

36. *Doctrine of Virtue*, 6:423.

37. 6:278–79.

38. "In this act [sex] a human being makes himself into a thing, which conflicts with the right of humanity in his own person." 6:278.

39. Similar points can also be made about Kant's discussion of self-enslavement at 6:283. See the discussion of both texts in D. Robert MacDougall, "Sometimes Merely as a Means: Why Kantian Philosophy Requires the Legalization of Kidney Sales," *The Journal of Medicine and Philosophy* 44, no. 3 (2019).

40. Katrin Flikschuh discusses the reasons that Kant's political philosophy requires a determination by the united will about what constitutes a person's body and criticizes Kant for thinking that we bear uncomplicated relationships to our bodies. See Katrin Flikschuh, "Innate Right and Acquired Right in Arthur Ripstein's Force and Freedom," *Jurisprudence* 1, no. 2 (2010). For an argument that defining Kantian body rights raises the same problems and requires the same (political) solutions as defining property rights, see Japa Pallikkathayil, "Persons and Bodies," in *Freedom and Force: Essays on Kant's Legal Philosophy*, ed. Sari Kisilevsky and Martin Jay Stone (Portland: Hart Publishing, 2017).

41. Ripstein, *Force and Freedom: Kant's Legal and Political Philosophy*, 135.

42. Translated from Latin, approximately: "to a willing person, injury is not done."

43. "Your body is the sum of your capacities to set and pursue your purposes." Ripstein, *Force and Freedom: Kant's Legal and Political Philosophy*, 40.

44. Ripstein, *Force and Freedom: Kant's Legal and Political Philosophy*, 142–43.

45. Ripstein, *Force and Freedom: Kant's Legal and Political Philosophy*, 140–41.

46. Ripstein, *Force and Freedom: Kant's Legal and Political Philosophy*, 136.

47. Ripstein, *Force and Freedom: Kant's Legal and Political Philosophy*, 133.

48. That persons can waive their rights is entailed by the fact that the *Doctrine of Right* argues only for an authorization (or right) to coerce, not for a duty to coerce. Kant earlier explicitly considered whether it was suitable to ground a theory of right in a doctrine of obligations; but he rejected the proposal precisely because it seemed absurd to hold that persons have a duty to enforce their own rights. See Immanuel Kant, "Review of Hufeland's Essay on the Principle of Natural Right," in *Practical Philosophy*, ed. and trans. Mary J. Gregor, The Cambridge Edition of the Works of Immanuel Kant (New York: Cambridge University Press, 1996), 8:129.

49. I assume that the organ becomes an individual's property; for a critical account of this assumption, see Pallikkathayil, "Persons and Bodies."

50. Barbara Cohen, "Surrogate Mothers: Whose Baby Is It?," *American Journal of Law & Medicine* 10, no. 3 (1984); Sara Ann Ketchum, "Selling Babies and Selling Bodies," *Hypatia* 4, no. 3 (1989).

Chapter 8

Legal Standards of Informed Consent and the Authority of the State

Bioethicists have, since the outset of the field, had much to say about the process of informed consent. One of the issues that has concerned them has been the amount of information physicians should be legally required to disclose in order to obtain informed consent. Several competing legal standards are currently in use and have been the object of a considerable amount of discussion by bioethicists. Courts have generally held physicians liable for disclosing either what physicians customarily disclose (the professional practice standard); what a reasonable patient would think material to the decision (the reasonable person standard); or what this particular patient would find material to the decision (the subjective standard).[1]

One of these standards—the professional practice standard, which regulates informed consent in about half of all U.S. states[2]—is a typical malpractice standard because it holds physicians accountable for disclosing what physicians customarily disclose. The other two standards, however, go beyond requiring mere conformity to the practices of other professionals. Both the reasonable person standard (the standard operative in the other half of U.S. states[3] and Canada) and the subjective standard (operative in the United Kingdom[4]) require disclosure of specific information about the risks and potential benefits—in other words, the consequences—of a proposed treatment, relative to its alternatives. These standards often require disclosing the likely consequences of patient decisions for a variety of outcomes, including survival, biological function, pain, comfort, lifestyle, psychology, and even social relationships. They also require informing patients about the relative likelihood and magnitude of the various consequences when these are known. These standards go beyond a duty to behave as a typical professional and instead impose what we might call a *duty to inform*. This legal duty to inform is a special duty insofar as it is not required of professionals when obtaining consent in most other contexts. Lawyers, car mechanics, engineers, financial advisers, and others all may have duties to inform clients about some specific risks or conflicts of interest, but they have no general obligation to inform clients about their options and the magnitude and likelihood of benefits and harms associated with each.

The claim that physicians and health researchers have a duty to obtain informed consent prior to treating or doing research first emerged in the context of research abuses.[5] The duty to inform is often treated as among researchers' and physicians' most stringent ethical duties. Bioethicists have, consequently, tried to ground this duty in the rights of patients, because rights are thought to be the most secure basis for such a stringent duty.

In this chapter I argue that bioethicists have failed to show that the duty to inform can be justified by direct appeal to patients' rights. They have failed because they haven't adequately attended to the limitations inherent in our prelegal rights, and have underestimated the important role that governments play in determining the character of our rights within a civil condition. By examining the implications of Kant's political philosophy for this issue, however, we can rectify this situation and justify a duty to inform in general and basic rights. The argument will proceed in three parts. First, I will show how bioethicists have tried to ground laws directly in general and basic rights—the kinds of rights that Kant argues we have in a state of nature, prior to and apart from a civil condition. But I will argue that none of the justifications succeeds, because general and basic rights are too general to ground the kinds of specific duties doctors supposedly have when obtaining informed consent. Then, I will argue that Kant anticipates this general problem in his political philosophy and suggests that the indeterminacy of basic rights is actually the main reason we must enter a civil condition: it is only within a civil condition, under a set of legitimate laws laid down by the state, that we can be fully equally free. I will argue that on the Kantian view, a duty to inform can be grounded ultimately in patients' rights, if the duty is imposed by a legitimate legal standard that can be understood as the product of a united will. I will argue that only some legal standards achieve this benchmark. Finally, I will argue that once the united will has laid down a legitimate standard for medical consent, that standard alters the moral duties of physicians, who have a duty to obey legitimate laws.

GENERAL AND BASIC RIGHTS TO CONSENT

Most authors have traced the justification for a duty to inform—ethical or legal—back to general and basic rights, as described by normative ethics theories. Rights capable of justifying a duty to inform need to be *general* in the sense that they are possessed by everyone. They could not simply be the rights created by a contract or specific promise, for example, because then a patient's right to be informed would depend on whether the patient had reached an understanding with a particular physician. The rights must further be *basic,* in the sense that they are prelegal. They cannot be rights created by law, because any such rights could not justify the laws on which they depend. Without prelegal moral rights, it would be difficult to criticize existing legal standards, which has long been an interest of bioethics. Here I consider three different accounts about how a duty to inform follows from basic and general rights. I argue that they all fail, because none has been able to reconcile physician's special duty to inform with patients' basic and general rights.

Autonomous Authorization

The most prominent moral justification for ethical and legal duties of disclosure is the *autonomous authorization* account, defended by Faden and Beauchamp[6] and Beauchamp and Childress.[7] On this account, the practices and standards surrounding informed consent are justified by their relationship to patient autonomy. An autonomous action, on their account, is one that is characterized by (among other things) "understanding." The understanding necessary for an autonomous action is a substantial understanding of the information material to the decision at hand, that is, whatever information the patient would consider "important" to the decision,[8] which generally includes understanding of the risks and potential benefits of a proposed intervention. Without this information, patients cannot understand and so cannot give autonomous authorizations. Because patients have a right to make autonomous decisions,[9] physicians must inform patients to obtain consent. Legal and ethical duties to inform are both justified in the same way, namely, by the fact that such duties are effective in producing autonomous authorizations.[10]

The autonomous authorization account can plausibly explain the special nature of the physician's duties to inform: it connects them directly to the patient's right to autonomy, which, on this account, requires that the patient understands the risks and benefits of treatment before making a decision. The problem for this account is that it simply isn't clear that patients have a moral right to this kind of autonomy. Certainly, it does not seem like such an autonomy right could be considered general and basic in the sense discussed earlier. If it was general and basic, one would think it would apply beyond the patient-physician relationship. But there is no general and basic right to be informed about the risks and benefits of one's decisions in other areas of life, such as getting married, going skydiving, eating deli meat, or having children, despite the fact that many of these have potential for large benefits or pose major risks.

In earlier versions of their work, Beauchamp and Childress made some attempt to root autonomy rights in the accounts of primary moral duties espoused by Kant and Mill.[11] There is no doubt that Kant and Mill both provide arguments in defense of a basic and general right to self-rule. But the problem with tracing informed consent to Kant or Mill is that it isn't clear that either theory requires being informed as a condition for the exercise of self-rule.[12] It would be surprising if either of these thinkers did support this: such a standard is not usually morally or legally required in any sort of decision other than medical decision making.

If there is no general and basic right to this kind of autonomy—and the autonomous authorization account provides no good reason for thinking there is—it is not clear that this account can show that physicians have a moral duty to inform at all.

Informed Consent as a Rights Waiver

Neil Manson and Onora O'Neill argue that instead of protecting autonomy, informed consent should be viewed as a waiver of a variety of rights one would otherwise have against health care professionals.[13] A full moral justification of informed consent consists, then, in an account of the various rights persons have against others (such as rights against coercion and deception, among other things) combined with an account about the circumstances under which persons can waive these rights.

Onora O'Neill develops an account of these rights and the duties to which they correspond.[14] O'Neill's account of "principled autonomy" draws its inspiration from Kantian moral philosophy. Essentially, principled autonomy requires persons to act on principles they could will everyone to act on.[15] To act autonomously, on this view, is to constrain one's actions so that they adhere to the basic tenets of practical reason. On this view, then, "autonomy" is a feature of actions (usually the actions of health care professionals or those who regulate or govern health care) that are constrained in the appropriate way, and is not a personal characteristic of patients or a reference to the authenticity of their choices.

O'Neill argues that various duties follow from principled autonomy, including negative duties to refrain from deception and coercion, as well as corresponding rights to be free of these things.[16] These duties and rights are the fundamental basis for the requirement to obtain informed consent,[17] as well as being the general basis for laws and policies that create a trustworthy society.[18]

O'Neill's account is attractive in part because rights not to be deceived or coerced seem both basic and general in a way that patients' rights to autonomy are not. As such this account could plausibly be thought morally to justify laws requiring consent. However, it is unclear why these general rights endow patients with a right to be informed about the consequences of their decisions. Even if one conceives the duty of nondeception very broadly, as O'Neill does (she claims it prohibits "lying, false promising, . . . manipulation. . .plagiarism" and more[19]), a positive right to be informed about the likely consequences of one's choices is not plausibly understood as entailed by the duty to avoid deception. This point is easily seen when we consider that a decision to engage in other kinds of similarly risky activities (such as mountaineering, boxing, or driving on the autobahn) without first being fully informed about the risks and benefits would not necessarily mean that the decision was the result of deception, even if others were present who knew about the risks.

O'Neill seems aware that there is a gap between very general duties like nondeception and the specific laws and policies governing informed consent. In response, she suggests that moral duties like nondeception function as very general moral constraints on the policies that can be chosen. Specific laws and policies governing consent in medicine should be chosen by considering a large variety of factors, including general moral constraints but also other kinds of practical matters and various nonmoral desiderata (for example, "clinical, scientific, financial, and technical constraints"[20]). However, if the duty to inform follows from such practical, nonmoral considerations, and not from the moral duties of noncoercion or nondeception themselves, then the problem remains unsolved. The rights-waiver view succeeds, perhaps, in justifying patients' rights to give bare consent, but fails to provide a distinctly moral rationale for the ethical or legal duty to inform associated with *informed* consent.

Fair Transactions

Miller and Wertheimer accept some elements of the autonomous authorization view but argue that an autonomous authorization is not ultimately necessary for successful consent transactions (that is, transactions that achieve what they call "moral transformation").[21] As they point out, consent transactions are often considered morally transformative even if one party or the other did not fully understand the consequences of the transaction. For example, when judging whether a contract is morally transformative, what is important is that the parties agree to the terms of the contract, not that they understand the consequences of signing the contract. The success of particular consent transactions cannot derive directly from consent, since consent is an internal state that can only be known with certainty by the agent him or herself.

For Miller and Wertheimer, consent transactions are morally transformative when both parties have a chance to token consent under "reasonably favorable" conditions. It is particularly important that neither party treats the other party "unfairly" during the transaction. While either party may be in a difficult situation, if both parties to the transaction act reasonably and fairly, the token of consent they give results in moral transformation.

Miller and Wertheimer's view is attractive in part because it offers an explanation about why requirements for medical consent differ from requirements for other kinds of consent: they differ because what counts as "fair" varies according to the context of the transaction. According to them, this means that treating a consenter "fairly" when agreeing to a sexual relationship differs significantly from treating a consenter "fairly" in a business transaction. In a medical transaction, information asymmetries generate unfairness between physician and patient, such that it would be unfair if the physician were to proceed without first fully informing the patient about the various benefits and risks of the proposed treatment.

However, Miller and Wertheimer give no explanation about fairness in general or about when imbalances between parties generate such special duties of fairness. Information asymmetries alone do not always generate a special duty to inform: as Miller and Wertheimer themselves discuss, if a long-term student of art history finds a painting that is significantly undervalued by its seller, it is not "unfair" for her to buy the painting without telling the seller what the painting is actually worth.[22] But if such information asymmetries are not unfair in art sales, what makes them unfair in the clinical context? Miller and Wertheimer give no further explanation. They seem to rely on intuitions or social conventions about fairness and unfairness in medical transactions when a moral argument is needed.

As I have stated, justifying physicians' duties to inform requires explaining why general and basic rights create heightened duties for physicians but not for professionals in nonmedical contexts. Miller and Wertheimer's account responds to the problem by positing a basic right to consent under fair conditions. If what is "fair" is highly context-dependent, as they claim, then perhaps this account can explain why medical standards might be idiosyncratic compared to the standards that are operative in nonmedical contexts. But without some general way of determining when a transaction is fair or unfair, it ultimately does not explain why fair transactions require physicians specifically to *inform* patients—rather than, for example, to offer them treatment at their own risk, under a caveat emptor standard, which also could constitute fairness in medical transactions. Miller and Wertheimer thus fail to justify informed consent because showing that it is possible that medical consent standards could be *different* from standards in other contexts is not yet to show that medical consent must be *informed*, where informed means understanding the possible consequences of one's decision.

The Problem with Appealing Directly to General and Basic Rights

I have argued so far that bioethicists have tried to defend ethical and legal duties to inform by appealing directly to general and basic rights. But this is problematic: general and basic rights might be the basis for general and basic duties, but it is unclear how physicians' special duties to inform could be derived from them. None of the accounts discussed so far has been able to bridge that gap satisfactorily. These accounts either defend special standards on the basis of putative rights that are not truly general and basic, like autonomy rights; or they defend them on the basis of general and basic rights, such as rights of nondeception, noncoercion, or fairness, that on closer examination do not specifically support a duty to inform.

The failure of such direct accounts is, I think, inevitable. The reason for this is bound up in what it would mean to justify special duties directly in general and basic rights. Let us say that a direct justification in general and basic rights would amount to a justification in those rights, without consideration of additional moral claims not strictly entailed by those rights. If special duties are distinguished from general duties in virtue of the fact that they are not entailed by general and basic rights, then special duties must necessarily rely on moral considerations beyond general and basic rights—in which case they would not be directly justified by these general and basic rights. For example, Miller and Wertheimer's fair transactions account stipulates that there is a general moral right to be treated fairly but claims that what counts as "fair" differs according to context. Even if we grant them this, they would need additional moral considerations beyond the general right to fairness in order to show why fairness requires a duty to inform in medicine. An account of the special moral requirements of fairness in medicine could provide this, but then their account would no longer ground special duties directly in general and basic rights, since it would make use of an auxiliary moral account of fairness in medicine.

Giving up on General and Basic Rights?

If general and basic rights cannot directly justify a special duty of disclosure, we might think it best to stop grounding the duty to inform in such rights altogether. Two different responses to such a failure may seem reasonable: we might conclude that a special duty to inform is not morally justifiable at all, or we might try to derive such a duty from some moral basis not ultimately appealing to rights, such as utilitarianism.

First, it might be tempting to conclude that there simply is no moral justification for ethical or legal duties to inform. General and basic rights can justify bare consent, and nothing more. Informed consent, and the laws aimed at protecting it, could be a medical custom with no substantive moral basis.

This conclusion should be accepted only hesitantly, and as a last resort, if no convincing moral justification can be found for ethical or legal duties to inform. Few if any ethical requirements are more strongly associated with physician ethics than informed consent. The fact that general and basic rights cannot easily be shown to ground the duty to inform does not by itself show that they cannot ground it all things considered.

If we continue searching for a moral justification for the duty to inform, a second strategy seems promising: perhaps the duty can be grounded in some alternative moral basis to general and basic rights, such as utility. Utility is, for example, arguably the ultimate ethical basis in accounts claiming to found physicians' special duties in information asymmetries.[23] The basic utilitarian argument for the duty to inform might go thus: information asymmetries between patients and physicians are an especially prominent feature of medicine, and either an ethical obligation or a public policy (or both) requiring physicians to remedy this asymmetry by informing patients will maximize utility in the long run.

This argument proceeds too quickly, however. First, even if we assume that information asymmetries are more prominent in medicine than in other fields, and even if we further assume that utility can only be maximized by eliminating or reducing such asymmetries, we would still need to show that the best way of reducing asymmetries is a law or ethical obligation requiring physicians to reduce it themselves by disclosing risks and potential benefits to patients. Information asymmetries are known in virtually every industry, but as already discussed, other industries do not solve the problem by simply requiring the more-informed party to systematically disclose the risks, potential benefits, and available options to the less-informed party. Instead, other mechanisms emerge to resolve such disparities. Those who purchase specialized services might become better educated about the product they buy, for example, by doing their own research, or they might utilize impartial consultants who are knowledgeable about the services or goods sought (such as potential homeowners do when they hire a home inspector). They might further gain insight into the competence and trustworthiness of specific physicians or practices by obtaining reviews written by experts (such as the reviews published in venues like *Consumer Reports* or the *Kelley Blue Book*) or those found on crowd-sourced websites (such as Zocdoc or Angie's List). In the absence of laws requiring disclosures, such venues would become more valuable and so more robust. A utilitarian justification of a duty to inform—whether legal or ethical—would need to show not merely that such a duty solves problems associated with information asymmetries, but also that it provides more utility than these other alternatives, all things considered.

I am not aware of any such utilitarian account, but even if one exists or could be given, it would likely raise a second problem: difficulty justifying the stringent ethical and legal duties usually associated with informed consent, which have been the object of wide consensus in bioethics. To illustrate this difficulty, consider James Stacey Taylor's argument that the ethical obligation of informed consent is best justified by appeal to patient well-being rather than respect for patient autonomy.[24] Taylor argues that informed consent cannot be based in respect for autonomy because failure to give a patient desired information could only be considered disrespect for patient autonomy in some cases, such as those involving intentional manipulation. Taylor argues that a duty to inform can instead be justified by its contribution to patient well-being: it puts patients in a better position to achieve their own preferences, and patients value having this information even when it doesn't.

However, as Taylor admits, justifying informed consent in terms of patient well-being makes the duty to inform conditional on a prior determination that informed consent is in the patient's interest. This weakens the case for either ethical or legal duties to inform relative to arguments based in patient rights. As Taylor concedes, if the well-being argument is accepted, "then the case for medical paternalism gains strength."[25]

This same problem is likely to accompany any effort to justify informed consent on the basis of something other than patient rights. The appeal of general and basic rights such as autonomy rights is, essentially, the unqualified nature of the duties associated with them. On such accounts, a patient's right to informed consent is not conditioned on any other values, and so is presumably stronger than those in which it is.

If a special duty to inform cannot be grounded directly in general and basic rights, and alternative ethical bases for this duty may not justify anything as stringent as an unqualified duty to obtain informed consent, then the problem remains unsolved. In what follows, I present an account that protects the stringency of informed consent requirements by giving them a foundation in general and basic rights. However, in order to solve the problem, I argue that the legal duty to inform is best understood to follow only *indirectly* from general and basic rights: general and basic rights form the ethical basis for a state with the authority to determine that special disclosures about the consequences of treatment are a necessary precondition for giving valid consent.

LEGAL STANDARDS FOR DISCLOSURE AND THE AUTHORITY OF THE STATE

Kant's political philosophy suggests a way of understanding why bioethicists' attempts to ground informed consent in general and basic rights have failed, and it also suggests a more plausible way of deriving a legal duty to inform from general and basic rights. In what follows, I will argue that the problem with existing justifications of the legal duty to inform is essentially the problem of indeterminacy in a state of nature. Kant solves the problem by arguing that our general and basic rights themselves do not directly solve the problem of indeterminacy; instead, they show the moral necessity of forming a state with the authority to determine the legal standards that will universally bind us, including legal standards determining what constitutes a valid consent to medical treatment.

Basic and General Rights in a State of Nature

As we saw in chapters 5 and 6, Kant—like the bioethicists we have so far surveyed—traces the moral basis of laws to general and basic rights. Kant's account starts with an account of our rights in a state of nature. In a state of nature persons have an innate right to freedom insofar as it can coexist with the freedom of everyone under universal law.

As I argued in chapter 7, innate right grounds a general right to enter into consensual relationships with others. Persons may consent to alter their duties and rights with respect to others by giving consent to alter them—in other words, by making a united choice. Because both rights to one's body and rights to one's property are within one's domain of freedom, one may waive any of those rights with respect to specific others by consenting. In cases where people make such a united choice to alter their respective freedoms, their choices are both necessary and sufficient for the alteration to be rightful. Because the choice does not, by definition, affect the rights of any nonconsenting parties, such uses of freedom can coexist with the freedom of everyone under universal law. This is the basic case for the right to sell one's organs, as I argued in chapter 7, and is also the basis for the right to consent to medical treatment.

The principle of innate right thus captures the central idea of a general and basic right of self-determination, and its correlative requirement of consent, that has been important both in bioethics and in the Western liberal tradition. Prior to any legislation or government, all persons have a right to give consent to others who would touch their bodies or to withhold it. Because this right is foundational it is an unconditional requirement, meaning that it serves as a side-constraint on all other politically permissible interactions. The Kantian view can thus explain the nonnegotiable and stringent nature of the duty to obtain consent before medical treatment. Such a duty is unconditional because it follows from the patient's innate right.

The Problem with the State of Nature

However, Kant recognized a problem with trying to specify any particular legal standard as following from this general and basic right to consent. This problem is a result of the indeterminacy of freedom under universal law. Many differing legal standards can effectively serve the purposes of ensuring that persons consent to treatment.

Kant explains this problem of indeterminacy in the context of property: to say that I have a *right* to some specific piece of property would be to unilaterally impose an obligation on everyone else not to interfere with it. But such unilateral imposition of obligation undermines the equal freedom of others. Without a set of laws that determines conclusively what belongs to each person by right and that is the object of a united and general will, the best I can do in a state of nature is to have provisional rights to things and to make rights claims that anticipate eventual ratification in a civil condition. Conclusive determination of the content of our rights is impossible in a state of nature because no one has the authority to unilaterally impose such claims on everyone else.

The same problem, as I noted in chapter 6, attends *any* free action in a state of nature. I cannot even enjoy a right to move freely because by claiming such a right I effectively unilaterally obligate all others to avoid the space I am in, which I have no right to do. This same problem attends interactions involving united choice, or bilateral interactions, such as those between a patient and physician. In a state of nature, neither party has fully determinate rights with respect to the other, even though each may have voluntarily entered the relationship. Although innate right establishes the necessity of consent, it leaves many other questions unanswered, even though answering these is instrumental to determining whether consent has occurred, and so when each is acting within their rights. To know when a consensual relationship is fully rightful, we would need to answer such questions as: Who is capable of giving consent? What must a person know, exactly, about a proposed interaction before he can give valid consent? Does consent to medical interventions require more disclosures than other kinds of interactions? If so, exactly how much disclosure is required? What signs indicate that a person has given consent? What must a person do to revoke consent? What kinds of actions—such as fraud or coercion—can undermine consent? And how are these to be defined?

Suppose that, in a state of nature, I contract with a physician for medical services. The physician proposes a treatment for my condition and tells me very little about any risks associated with the treatment. I assume, though, that if there were any major risks, she would have explained these. I consent to and undergo the operation but, through no fault of the physician, I suffer a significant harm. I suppose that, if I had known about the risk of harm, I would not have undergone the procedure. I contact the physician to request that she compensate me for the damages I have incurred, which are significant. I suppose that I have a provisional right to be informed about any such significant harm, otherwise my consent is invalid. But she refuses to compensate me because she supposes she has a provisional right to offer medical treatment without informing me about major risks. She supposes that if I would have liked to know about the risks, I could have asked her or could have sought further information on my own. Essentially, I believe that I have a right to be informed, and she believes that I do not. Let us assume, for the moment, that either right could serve as a universal law, making us both equally free. Unfortunately, we have different and mutually incompatible understandings of the content of our provisional rights in a state of nature.

In this situation in a state of nature, I am authorized to force her to pay damages because she has violated my provisional rights. However, she is also authorized to employ force to resist my attempts to collect compensation: by approaching her with force, I am violating her provisional rights. Neither one of us is required to defer to the other's understanding of provisional rights. If one of us were required to defer to the other's understanding, it would make the two of us unequal, and so would violate innate right. Whoever is most capable of enforcing their own understanding of provisional rights will be able to protect their own freedom, so much the worse for the other. This situation illustrates the tragedy of the state of nature. Neither of us acts specifically wrongly, but we do each other a great wrong overall insofar as we refuse to enter with each other into a civil condition, where our freedom can be made equal under universal law. In a state of nature, there is no way of resolving rights disputes, and so we inevitably wrong others (as they do us) when we choose to remain without a law or mechanism for resolving the rightful bounds of the freedom of each.

The Kantian discussion of the indeterminacy of rights in a state of nature helps further explain why bioethicists' justifications of informed consent have failed. They have failed because they have tried to ground duties to inform directly in patients' general and basic rights. But although consent itself is required in order to preserve the equal freedom of each, in a state of nature it is not clear exactly when consent has been produced. It could be that valid consent has not been obtained until the patient has been fully informed about the risks and benefits material to the current decision. On the other hand, it is also possible that valid consent can occur even when the patient has not been informed at all about likely benefits or risks of the treatment. Either could serve as a universal law in a state of nature. The tragedy is that, without someone to conclusively settle what constitutes a valid consent, each person is entitled to decide for herself what she considers to be a valid consent, in accordance with the rule she thinks would be adopted in a civil condition. Both doctors and patients have the authority to determine the provisionally rightful nature of a valid consent. But as we have seen, although a presumption about what one is authorized to do with respect to others is morally necessary in a state of nature, such presumptions inevitably lead to a state of violence, when the presumptions of each about the content of our respective rights bump up against the presumptions of others.

The Civil Condition as the Solution to the Problem

As we saw in chapter 6, the problem of violence can be solved by moving from a state of nature into a civil condition. Entering a civil condition with others means agreeing with them to be governed under the institutions of the state: a legislator, an executive, and a judiciary. The laws passed in such a condition do not represent unilateral wills but rather an omnilateral will. So they do not amount to unilateral imposition of obligations. As we saw in chapter 6, there is a duty to enter such a civil condition because it is the only way to preserve the equal freedom of each under universal law.

The state can also solve the problem of differing standards or ideas about what constitutes a valid consent to medical treatment. By laying down a single legal standard that binds everyone, it makes clear precisely what physicians must disclose to patients in order for any subsequent consent to treatment to be considered valid.

Potentially, then, the state can choose some legal standard endowing physicians with a duty to inform, and can require that physicians meet this standard as a condition for obtaining valid consent. If so, then Kant effectively explains how a duty to inform can be grounded in basic and general rights. Innate right—the right to freedom that can coexist with the freedom of everyone—entails the necessity of consent in a state of nature. However, determining what exactly is required for a valid consent to medical treatment is not directly resolved by innate right: there are many ways of making persons free of others under universal law, because there are multiple mutually exclusive candidates for universal laws governing medical consent. To be equally free, we need to enter into a civil condition and submit to a state that can lay down a conclusive law determining what, exactly, is required for valid consent to medical treatment. Once this standard has been laid down, it stipulates what is actually required for consent, and violating the law is tantamount to violating the equal freedom of others, since protecting the equal freedom of everyone is the purpose for which the state and its laws exists. So, if the state endows physicians with a legal duty to inform, then they must inform patients before treating them; treating a patient without informing him will fail in obtaining his consent and so infringes on his equal freedom under universal law.

Laws and Their Limits in a Civil Condition

However, before we accept this conclusion, we need to determine whether either of the proposed "duty to inform" standards for physicians' disclosures discussed at the beginning of the chapter could legitimately be implemented by the state. I noted earlier that several competing legal standards for medical consent are used in different jurisdictions. Two of these (the reasonable person standard and the subjective standard) endow physicians with a duty to inform, because they impose a legal duty on physicians to disclose specific information about risks and benefits. Could either of these "duty to inform" standards be legitimate regulations of medical disclosures?

It may seem, initially, that the answer to this question is "yes." In chapter 6 I argued that the most general limitation on laws in a civil condition is that they must serve to maintain the freedom of all, which is to say they must limit freedom only for the purpose of ensuring the freedom of others. This is the general test for whether a law could be the object of a united will, because persons have no duty to agree to any law that limits their freedom for any other purpose. Since standards for consent exist precisely for the purpose of determining *when consent is valid*, it may seem that both "duty to inform" standards fulfill the overall purpose of law, namely, ensuring that each party is free of the other, since consent is the most general means of maintaining our freedom.

However, it is important not only that a legal standard ostensibly serves the purpose of making each person equally free, but also that it does so in a manner that preserves the equal freedom of each. In other words, laws cannot legitimately make persons subservient to one another, even if they supposedly do so for the purpose of ensuring equal freedom. One way of testing this is by asking whether each citizen individually could consent to the laws as a means of ensuring their equal freedom. I will argue that when we subject each of the "duty to inform" standards to this test of legitimacy, we can see that the reasonable person standard is legitimate but that the subjective standard is not.

Legitimacy and Duty to Inform Standards

The Reasonable Person Standard

The reasonable person standard, as we said earlier, requires the physician to disclose all the information that a hypothetical reasonable person would find material to the decision. This standard does fulfill the basic purpose of law. We can see how by examining first how it limits the freedom of both parties and then by showing how those limits serve the purpose of preserving the freedom of others.

The reasonable person standard limits the freedom of each party by defining the conditions under which consent is valid. The physician is limited in the sense that she may consider the patient to have given valid consent only if she has disclosed information up to the level required by the standard—that is, up to the level that a reasonable person would think material to the decision. The patient's freedom, likewise, is limited in the sense that he must consider valid any consent he gave to a physician who fully provided this level of disclosure. He may not claim that his consent was invalid because the physician did not give him some piece of information he later decides he would have liked to have, for example.

These limitations stand in contrast to the total lack of limitations in a state of nature. In a state of nature, either party could make a provisionally rightful claim that the other party did not fully satisfy its rights, regardless of what the other party actually did, because there is no single universal standard laid down determining when a valid consent has been given. But once a standard like the reasonable person standard is laid down in a civil condition, the freedom of each party to a medical interaction is limited: each may complain about a rights violation only in the case that the other does not perform what is required by the standard.

Although the reasonable person standard limits the freedom of each party, it does so for the purpose of preserving the freedom of the other. The limits on the patient serve to preserve the freedom of the physician: the physician knows that so long as she has met the objective standards for disclosure required by law, she has performed her legal duty and has not violated the patient's rights, even if the patient did not get as much information as he would have liked. The limits on the physician serve to preserve the freedom of the patient: the patient knows that the physician will disclose all the information that a reasonable person would find material to the decision, and the patient will have legal recourse in the case that it turns out that the physician does not achieve this standard. Because the standard is objective, both physician and patient can determine independently that they are complying with the rights of the other party. Both parties can make a free choice about whether to participate in the medical intervention, knowing in advance what this will mean for their respective rights. The judgment about whether participation will further their own individual ends is up to each party to judge for themselves.

Because the reasonable person standard can be understood as limiting freedom of each to uphold the equal freedom of others, it could be the object of a united and general will. Consequently, the reasonable person standard can be understood as a legitimate legal standard on the Kantian theory. We can conclude, then, that the Kantian argument succeeds where other theories have failed to show how basic and general rights justify a duty to inform, at least in those jurisdictions employing a reasonable person standard.

The Subjective Standard and the Limits of Legitimacy

Not all standards requiring physicians to inform are similarly justifiable on the Kantian view, however. The subjective standard differs in important respects from the reasonable person standard, and on at least one interpretation could not be considered legitimate, even if it were chosen through the normal political process within a civil condition.

On the subjective standard, the adequacy of the information given to the patient is determined by whether it constitutes the information that is "material" to the particular patient,[26] that is, the information that is important to the patient, given his or her ends or values. The subjective standard thus makes the adequacy of the physician's disclosure and the resulting consent a function of the patient's ends. In contrast, the reasonable person standard is an objective standard because the standard for disclosure does not depend on the ends of either party. This shift away from an objective standard determined independently of either party to a subjective standard determined by the ends of one party creates three problems[27] with respect to the united and general will.

First, by making the physician accountable to the patient's *ends,* the subjective standard construes the relationship as one in which one private party (the physician) has a duty to aid or help another (the patient) achieve his or her goals or ends, such that the patient cannot give a valid consent to treatment unless the physician offers the required assistance toward the patient's individual aims. This goes beyond the justifiable rationale for law: on the Kantian argument, the purpose of laws is to achieve the freedom of each party, and the only possible basis for limiting one party's freedom of choice is to preserve the freedom of choice of the other. Individuals do not have a fundamental or innate right to receive help in achieving their ends; innate right is instead freedom from others. Nor do individuals have fundamental legal duties to assist others, but only to preserve others' freedom. Because laws limiting one person's freedom to help another achieve his or her ends are not consistent with the primary rationale of law, which is to preserve the freedom of each, they are such that free and equal persons could not agree to them.

Second, by making the ends of only one party legally significant, the subjective standard necessarily makes the parties unequal. As noted above, the subjective standard makes the validity of consent dependent on whether the information disclosed was all the information that the patient wanted, that is, the information that the patient finds useful for achieving his ends. The standard does not reference the ends of the physician, however, and the reason is obvious: a legal standard could make rightfulness a function of the ends of one party, at most, because parties can have different or even mutually exclusive ends. The validity of consent could not depend, for example, on the information that the patient wants to receive *as well as* the information that the physician wants to give. The kind of disclosure the parties find conducive to their personal ends could be different, and if it was different, there would be no way to determine whether the resulting consent was valid. Because the patient's ends determine the rightfulness of the transaction in a way that the physician's do not, the subjective standard makes the parties unequal. In contrast, objective standards such as the reasonable person standard do not make rightfulness a function of the ends of either party, but only whether the actions of each conform to the external standard; as such, objective standards preserve the equality of both parties.

Third, by making the satisfaction of the physician's legal duty dependent on the patient's ends, the subjective standard essentially permits the patient to determine the law for the physician. Innate right, says Kant, is a right to freedom or "independence from constraint by the choice of another." The subjective standard does not give the patient the right to directly constrain the physician, but the patient does have power to indirectly constrain the choice of the physician, insofar as the patient has the authority to determine the legal standard to which the physician is held. Objective standards do not raise this problem: even if the standard requires different amounts of effort or places different burdens on the parties, the legal rights of neither party are *determined* by the other party to the transaction. The subjective standard, however, legally instantiates a relationship of subjection between interacting parties. On Kant's view, this runs directly counter to the purpose of law, which is to make private parties independent of each other.

Most commentators criticizing the subjective standard have argued that the major problem with it is an epistemic one: the physician cannot know whether she has given the patient all the information he would like to know.[28] Other standards also raise epistemic problems, however. The reasonable person standard requires the physician to judge what a reasonable person would want to know, but this standard is vague, and the findings of juries in particular cases are thus somewhat unpredictable. Similarly, the professional practice standard requires disclosure of whatever physicians customarily disclose, but accurate information about the customs of other physicians may be unavailable to the physician and/or patient or even nonexistent. Epistemic problems are not restricted to the subjective standard, and such criticisms seem to accompany any of the competing standards.

The Kantian view is useful for showing why the main problem with the subjective standard is not epistemic but relational. Because the subjective standard makes the physician's rights and duties a function of the patient's subjective ends, it undermines the physician's freedom, makes the patient and physician unequal, and makes the individual patient lawgiver to the physician. The subjective standard is thus a law that a people could not will for itself. Any justifiable legal standard must, on the Kantian view, be an objective one that both parties can independently choose to meet, rather than a subjective one that gives one party legal control over the rightfulness of the other's actions.

On a different interpretation of the subjective standard, however, some of these problems may be avoided. As Beauchamp and Childress qualify this standard, it requires disclosure of information material to the particular patient only insofar as "it is reasonable to expect the physician to determine the patient's informational needs."[29] The crucial point here is who determines what counts as "reasonable." If "reasonable" is understood as "reasonable from the point of view of the patient," then the standard does not meaningfully preserve the freedom and equality of the physician, as discussed above. If, on the other hand, "reasonable" is determined by what most other prudent physicians would do to determine the patient's needs, or by what most reasonable people would do to determine the patient's needs, then the subjective standard is actually an objective standard because the standard for disclosure is not set directly by either party's ends.

However, note that these "objective" interpretations of the subjective standard would serve partially to undermine the main argument for adopting the subjective standard in the first place, which is its supposed value for preserving patient autonomy.[30] If patients have a right only to a physician who makes a reasonable attempt to determine their needs, where "reasonable" is determined according to some standard independent and outside of the patient, then the ability of the patient to exercise autonomy by making decisions based on completely individualized or idiosyncratic preferences is effectively undermined. Patients are not then entitled to all the information they want (or would want, if they knew what the physician knew), but only to what someone else could reasonably guess they would want.

ETHICS AND THE LAW

I have argued thus far that patients can have a conclusive right to information from physicians, and physicians can have a duty to inform patients, if and only if there is a legitimate legal standard requiring as much. The reasonable person standard can be such a legitimate standard because it is objective and thus ensures the equal freedom of both patients and physicians. The legal standard effectively determines the specific nature and content of our general and basic rights to freedom.

If this is so, then it seems that the relevant legal standards not only determine our legal rights with respect to each other, but they also determine our moral duties, at least to some extent. As I argued in chapter 6, legitimate laws impose political obligations on us; the civil condition is necessitated by the fact that it is only way of fully respecting others' rights to freedom under universal law. Consequently, the laws that emerge out of a civil condition are obligatory because they are just the specification of the more general duty not to violate others' rights. Physicians consequently have not only a legal duty to meet the relevant legal standards, they also have a moral one.

Because we now have an account of physicians' duties and patients' rights in a civil condition, it is also possible to explain the specific character of physicians' moral duties to honor the Categorical Imperative when obtaining consent. In chapter 6 I argued that acting in ways against which others have rights necessarily *uses* them, and so requires consent. So, taking someone else's money uses *them*, and requires consent if it is to avoid treating that person merely as a means. Acting in ways against which others have no rights, however, may merely affect them. Rights thus play a crucial role in determining whether an action necessarily uses someone.

The same basic reasoning determines the character of the physician's duty to use patients as ends, and not merely as a means, when obtaining informed consent. In jurisdictions that have adopted a legitimate "duty to inform" standard, such as those that have adopted the reasonable person standard, physicians must conform to the relevant legal standard in order to ensure that they use their patients as ends, and not merely as a means. This is because patients in these jurisdictions have a right to be informed about the benefits and risks of treatment as a condition for giving valid consent. If physicians use patients without first disclosing the benefits and risks that a reasonable person would want to know, physicians act in ways against which patients have rights, and so *use* them. On the other hand, if no "duty to inform" standard is in place—for example, in jurisdictions with a professional practice standard—then failing to inform patients about the risks and benefits of treatment may *affect* the patients but does not necessarily use them. Consequently, informing patients in these jurisdictions is not strictly necessary for ensuring that one does not use them as a mere means.[31] So in this case, we can see how the specification of the relevant legal standard affects not just the legal duties of physicians, but also their moral duties. The law determines what belongs to each by right, and so determines when treating patients as ends requires informing them.

Two qualifications are important here. First, just as it is generally possible to use someone as an end by securing their consent to something that would otherwise violate their rights, patients may consent to relieve physicians of their duty to inform. This is just a right to waive one's right to be informed about benefits and risks. So, even in duty to inform jurisdictions physicians have no legal or moral duty to inform patients about benefits and risks if patients do not want them to.[32] Patients would, however, have to make clear in a legally recognizable manner that they understood they had a right to be informed and that they were accepting legal responsibility for waiving this right.

Second, informing patients to the extent required by law does not guarantee that patients are used as ends rather than merely as a means. If a physician knows, for example, that some particular piece of information that is not legally required would be extremely important to a patient's decision even though it is not legally required (because, for example, most reasonable persons would not want to know it) but withholds that information simply in order to frustrate the patient, then the physician use the patient as a mere means. As I argued in chapter 6, the law provides something like a floor for what we may morally do to one another: by violating someone's legal rights, we necessarily use them as a mere means. This does not guarantee that if we respect their legal rights that we necessarily use them as ends in themselves. Whether we fully satisfy the requirement to treat someone as an end in herself depends on the precise reason for which we act, specifically whether we make the other person's ends our own. So conforming with our legal duties does not exhaust our moral duties even though obeying the law is morally required.

In chapter 1, I argued that it is impossible to make adequate recommendations about the ethics of clinical practice unless one understands whether laws have the ability to alter or determine the nature of these duties. For example, it is impossible to say whether it is ethically permissible to assist in a patient's suicide in jurisdictions that prohibit assisted suicide, unless one has an account about whether laws can impose moral obligations on us. Now we can see in more detail how political philosophy can help us determine the moral obligations of clinicians. If, as I have argued, legitimate laws can impose moral obligations on us, then physicians have a moral duty to obey those laws, even if those laws require something that would not clearly otherwise be their moral duty.[33] In this case, if laws endow physicians with a legal duty to inform their patients about the risks and benefits of treatment, then physicians have a moral duty to inform their patients, even if there is no definitive way of showing they would have such a moral duty in a state of nature.

BIOETHICS AND THE PROMISE OF NORMATIVE POLITICAL PHILOSOPHY

This discussion of the implications of Kant's political philosophy for legal standards of disclosure helps to show both a general problem with the typical bioethics approach, and the promise of normative political philosophy for bioethics. Long-standing problems in bioethics, such as the question about which legal standards should govern informed consent, exist in part because bioethics employs the wrong tools to solve them. Bioethicists have insisted on solving these problems by referring only to general and basic rights, but these have not been able to justify any specific laws about physicians' duties or patients' rights, because general and basic rights by themselves are not determinate enough to establish laws governing medical practice. In order to determine which laws we should have in a civil condition, we need an account not just of general and basic rights, but also an account about how the government can or should go about securing these. What we need, in other words, is an account of what makes government good or just or legitimate. It is only then that we will have a reasonably adequate account about which legal standards of disclosure to choose.

A political view—or at least, a Kantian one—can go some of the way in correcting this problem with bioethics. The Kantian political view I have offered here connects an account of general and basic rights with an account of government legitimacy: if we have an innate right to be free, then laws will be legitimate only if they serve the purpose of instantiating that freedom. Even laws that determine our rights and duties with more specificity than is possible in a state of nature can be legitimate because they are arrived at through the procedures established in the civil condition for protecting our equal freedom. The theory of legitimacy can help us distinguish between legitimate legal standards (such as the reasonable person standard) and illegitimate ones (such as the subjective standard). When the state imposes a legitimate legal standard endowing physicians with a duty to inform, such as the reasonable person standard, then physicians really do have a duty to inform patients, and patients have a corresponding right to be informed. Patients' rights to be informed, moreover, are ultimately based in their general and basic rights, because innate right endows them with a right to have the specific content of their rights laid down conclusively in a civil condition. Consequently, in jurisdictions employing a "duty to inform" standard, patients have an unconditional right to be informed before medical treatment, just as physicians have a stringent duty to inform them.

Incidentally, by specifying the legal obligations of physicians when obtaining consent, the Kantian political view also helps us to specify the moral floor for physician behaviors. This is because the political view tells us when laws are morally binding. If physicians are required by a legitimate legal standard to disclose whatever a reasonable person would want to know and the patient has not waived his right to this, then physicians who do not meet this legal requirement necessarily use patients as mere means. Without an explanation of when laws can be morally binding on physicians, there is no way to know whether physicians who fail to fulfill their legal duties also violate their moral ones. The political view, then, can also solve a second problem that bioethicists working on informed consent have not yet tried to solve:[34] it can tell us how existing laws alter the moral obligations of physicians. If giving all-things-considered ethical advice to physicians is a task of clinical bioethics, then here we can see another reason for bringing the tools of political philosophy into bioethics.

NOTES

1. Tom L. Beauchamp and James F. Childress, *Principles of Biomedical Ethics*, 7th ed. (New York: Oxford University Press, 2013), 125–27.

2. David M. Studdert et al., "Geographic Variation in Informed Consent Law: Two Standards for Disclosure of Treatment Risks," *Journal of Empirical Legal Studies* 4, no. 1 (2007).

3. Studdert et al., "Geographic Variation in Informed Consent Law: Two Standards for Disclosure of Treatment Risks."

4. Daniel K. Sokol, "Update on the UK Law on Consent," *British Medical Journal* 350 (2015).

5. The first statement of ethics making reference to a duty of *informed* consent was the Declaration of Helsinki (1964), which is widely recognized as building on the Nuremberg Code (1947), responding to the abuses of Nazi physicians (Robert V. Carlson, Kenneth M. Boyd, and David J. Webb, "The Revision of the Declaration of Helsinki: Past, Present and Future.," *British Journal of Clinical Pharmacology* 57, no. 6 [2004].). In the United States, duties of researchers to obtain informed consent were posited in the *Belmont Report* (1978), which was formed in part to respond to the abuses of the Tuskegee Syphilis Study. Physicians' legal duties to obtain informed consent developed in the United States in the context of case law, but are widely thought to be required for the same ethical reasons that informed consent is required in research on human subjects.

6. Ruth R. Faden and Tom L. Beauchamp, *A History and Theory of Informed Consent* (New York: Oxford University Press, 1986).

7. Beauchamp and Childress, *Principles of Biomedical Ethics*, 7th ed.
8. Faden and Beauchamp, *A History and Theory of Informed Consent*, 302–4.
9. Beauchamp and Childress, *Principles of Biomedical Ethics*, 7th ed., 107.
10. Faden and Beauchamp, *A History and Theory of Informed Consent*, 284.
11. Tom L. Beauchamp and James F. Childress, *Principles of Biomedical Ethics*, 5th ed. (New York: Oxford University Press, 2001), 63–64.
12. Sigurdur Kristinsson, "Autonomy and Informed Consent: A Mistaken Association?," *Medicine, Health Care and Philosophy* 10, no. 3 (2007). He capably explains why Kantian ethics could not justify informed consent. He does however find in Mill arguments supporting the positive value of informed deliberation and argues that these could be taken as reasons for supporting something like a duty to inform. Mill however never made this argument (as Kristinsson admits), and it strains the imagination to think that if he had, he would support such duties only for medical decision making.
13. Neil C. Manson and Onora O'Neill, *Rethinking Informed Consent in Bioethics* (Cambridge: Cambridge University Press, 2007), 72–77.
14. Onora O'Neill, *Autonomy and Trust in Bioethics* (Cambridge: Cambridge University Press, 2003).
15. O'Neill, *Autonomy and Trust in Bioethics*, 84.
16. O'Neill focuses on duties, not rights, but suggests in numerous instances that she sees patient rights as correlatives to physicians' duties to avoid coercion and deception. For example, see O'Neill, *Autonomy and Trust in Bioethics*, 95.
17. O'Neill, *Autonomy and Trust in Bioethics*, 97.
18. O'Neill, *Autonomy and Trust in Bioethics*, 123.
19. O'Neill, *Autonomy and Trust in Bioethics*, 98.
20. O'Neill, *Autonomy and Trust in Bioethics*, 125.
21. Franklin G Miller and Alan Wertheimer, "Preface to a Theory of Consent Transactions: Beyond Valid Consent," in *The Ethics of Consent: Theory and Practice*, ed. Franklin G. Miller and Alan Wertheimer (Oxford: Oxford University Press, 2010); "The Fair Transaction Model of Informed Consent: An Alternative to Autonomous Authorization," *Kennedy Institute of Ethics Journal* 21, no. 3 (2011).
22. Miller and Wertheimer, "Preface to a Theory of Consent Transactions: Beyond Valid Consent," 95.
23. Arrow argued that many of the special features of the organization of medicine can be explained as economically rational responses to information asymmetries. But as Arrow himself admits, there is more than one economically rational way of dealing with information asymmetries. Kenneth Arrow, "Uncertainty and the Welfare Economics of Medical Care," *The American Economic Review* 53, no. 5 (1963).
24. James Stacey Taylor, "Autonomy and Informed Consent: A Much Misunderstood Relationship," *The Journal of Value Inquiry* 38, no. 3 (2005).
25. Taylor, "Autonomy and Informed Consent: A Much Misunderstood Relationship," 391.
26. Faden and Beauchamp, *A History and Theory of Informed Consent*, 33.
27. My discussion of the three problems is structured around Kant's three "attributes of a citizen": freedom, equality, and independence (6:314).

28. Beauchamp and Childress, *Principles of Biomedical Ethics*, 7th ed., 127; Vilius Dranseika, Jan Piasecki, and Marcin Waligora, "Relevant Information and Informed Consent in Research: In Defense of the Subjective Standard of Disclosure," *Science and Engineering Ethics* 23, no. 1 (2016).

29. Beauchamp and Childress, *Principles of Biomedical Ethics*, 7th ed., 127.

30. Beauchamp and Childress, *Principles of Biomedical Ethics*, 7th ed., 127; Dranseika, Piasecki, and Waligora, "Relevant Information and Informed Consent in Research: In Defense of the Subjective Standard of Disclosure."

31. Since the duty to inform is determined in these jurisdictions by the customary practices of other physicians, it is not *necessarily* the case that physicians will always have a duty to inform because their duties in such cases are contingent on the activities of other physicians. If it is customary for physicians to inform patients about the relevant procedure in these jurisdictions then, obviously, the patient will have a right to be informed and physicians will also have both a moral and legal duty to inform.

32. This is sometimes treated as the "problem of waivers" in bioethics. See Beauchamp and Childress, *Principles of Biomedical Ethics*, 7th ed., 137. On Kant's view, waivers of even fundamental rights—such as rights against having one's own kidneys removed, as we saw in chapter 7—must be possible, because prohibiting such waivers effectively gives some third party the authority to decide what use a patient will make of his own freedom. Although Beauchamp and Childress claim that waivers of informed consent are potentially dangerous, it is difficult to see why they are more problematic than other kinds of rights waivers which everyone accepts. If patients can waive their rights not to be cut open for the purpose of surgery or can waive their right not to be subject to potentially dangerous research, then they can presumably also waive their right to be informed about the benefits and risks of a particular treatment.

33. This is not to imply that laws prohibiting assisted suicide are legitimate under the Kantian view; they likely would not be, for the same reason laws prohibiting organ sales are not.

34. As far as I'm aware. Bioethicists don't typically treat the question about the moral obligatoriness of laws because the field is so heavily predisposed toward thinking of primary moral duties as the basis for, rather than the result of, laws.

Conclusion

When the Presidential Council on Bioethics was formed during George W. Bush's presidency, American bioethics underwent a profound self-examination. This self-examination was occasioned by the fact that the Council included many bioethicists who were not on the left end of the political spectrum, thus breaking with a long-standing pattern of appointing left-leaning bioethicists to governmental bodies.[1] Bioethicists were widely critical of the Bush Council. They worried that the Council would "politicize" bioethics.

At first glance, it is difficult to understand the scandal caused by the appointment of the Bush Council. As various commentators pointed out, the Council was likely the most politically diverse commission that had ever been appointed; previous presidents had made no effort to reflect the political diversity of the electorate.[2] Moreover, conservative bioethicists were no new phenomenon. Bioethicists had been quietly divided about issues such as abortion and genetic technologies since the beginning of the field.[3] The Council was appointed by a Republican president, for the purposes of his own advisement; presidents undoubtedly have the right to appoint anyone they wish to advise them. The Council would have no official power. Their first charge was not to make a decision about any particular policy, but to "undertake fundamental inquiry into the human and moral significance of developments in biomedical and behavioral science and technology."[4] The Council was further given permission to choose whether to issue consensus positions or to reflect a diversity of views.[5] Although many worried about the impact the Council would have on embryonic stem cell research policy—a subject of intense national debate at the time—the President appointed the Council the same day he announced his decision to limit funding for federal stem cell research. Why did bioethicists care about the membership of such a council?

The controversy caused by the appointment of the Council is best understood by examining the history of the field. As we saw in chapter 2, major methods of bioethics had been conceived specifically for the purpose of reconciling pluralistic outlooks on morality. The *Belmont Report* had found three mid-level principles, widely shared in our culture; Beauchamp and Childress had found four principles that they claimed represented the common morality, universally shared among morally serious persons. Other bioethicists after them had proposed alternative methods for bioethics, also premised around the idea of finding some basis for consensus: principles or rules that could be widely accepted as the basis for shared decisions in a pluralistic context. On some accounts, bioethics owed its success in influencing policy in part to the fact that it was not obviously partisan.[6]

Bioethicists reacted to the appointment of a politically divided council in part because they predicted (correctly) that a politically divided commission working on politically divisive issues would draw attention to the controversial nature of the policy recommendations that bioethicists had been making for quite some time. The entrance of conservative bioethicists to such a prominent bioethics body gave an unmistakable signal: issues in bioethics would now have to be conceived of as subject to the same kinds of polarization and politicization that characterize other public debates. The days of asserting conclusions on the basis of consensus, widely shared by persons on all sides of the political spectrum, were over.

Those days seem ever more distant now. It is important to say why they are over. One of the reasons has to do with the way that political cultures have evolved in an age of social media and information overload. Political partisanship, polarization, and distrust are at an all-time high. It is unlikely that any set of principles can cut through the noise and unify us at this point.

But Bush's Council also revealed a second reason why the days of the old approach to policy are over: the old methods were never adequate to begin with. One thing that became apparent at the time of the Bush Council was that the theories and principles in use by previous commissions were actually doing very little work; the appearance of consensus within prior commissions had more to do with the members selected for those groups, the homogeneity of their politics, and their agreement to avoid controversial issues, than it did with the application of a theory capable of representing our shared values, such as the principles of the *Belmont Report*. The principles, as a method for justifying policy recommendations, worked fine until those applying them had serious disagreements. At that point, law and policy recommendations supposedly issuing from a "common morality" quickly wore thin because they looked like they sought to enforce an unshared morality.

As we saw in chapter 2, proponents of principles based in a common morality, such as Beauchamp and Childress, have no theoretical defense against charges of "enforcing morality" because their work implicitly assumes that morality *should* be enforced, and that any moral norm that is part of the common morality could be a suitable basis for law and policy, perhaps with some pragmatic exceptions. The best defense for the enforcement of these moral norms is that they are *common*. But when the sense of common values breaks down, recommendations based on common values lose their perceived legitimacy.

Bioethics is now irretrievably politicized, for better or worse, but the loss of apparent consensus also makes it possible for us to depart from the old methods of consensus bioethics and ask: can we do better? If we aren't constrained to follow the three principles of Belmont, the four principles of Beauchamp and Childress, or some other set of principles designed to form a consensus suitable as a basis for public policy, then how might we improve on the methods that have come to characterize bioethics' treatment of law and policy?

Most importantly, bioethics should take up political philosophy and make normative recommendations based on a vision about what makes government just or legitimate or good. In this book I have illustrated how this might work and why it is important. Kant's view, I have explained, makes a principled distinction between moral duties that are the responsibilities of individuals, and the rights claims that we may legitimately impose on others. In this way, the Kantian view does not face charges of "enforcing morality" in the same way that the variety of bioethics theories we examined do. Kant's theory could, I think, stand up better in a pluralistic age than theories that depend on the idea that we share some underlying morality. This is because Kant's view assumes we have different, even radically different, ends and that the role of the government is to make us free and equal but not to guarantee some specific outcome that necessarily only represents some views about the good. Other political theories are, to varying extents, similar in this regard. By presenting a vision of what makes government good or just or legitimate—instead of just a vision of what makes human conduct good, as bioethics theories typically have presented—political theories generally find it reasonable to distinguish between the primary rights and duties that bind everyone, and the secondary rights and duties that are more directly applicable to governments. This may lead to a vision of government that looks something like Mill's classically liberal government, or Rawls's politically liberal one. What these theories share with Kantian deontological liberalism is the idea that there are norms specifically applicable to governments, and that these norms are based on considerations other than enforcement of moral duty.

Regardless of whether it is right to say that, in a pluralistic age, Kant's view is more widely acceptable than ideas of common morality, there is a second, less speculative advantage enjoyed by Kant's theory over existing methods in bioethics: Kant's political philosophy is conceptually capable of justifying law and policy. Failure in this regard is the main problem, I have argued, with the methods of bioethics. Bioethicists have always wanted to justify law and policy but have rarely even acknowledged the conceptual difference between showing the existence of a moral duty and showing the legitimacy of enforcing one. What we need is overt attention to the question about what makes government just or legitimate or good. Until we have an account of this, we do not have arguments for laws and policies at all.

Kant provides an account about the legitimacy of government. On his account, legitimacy is a function of our right to be externally free of others under universal law. His account is a sufficient basis from which to make political judgments about health policy and law, as I have illustrated in this book. But as I noted in the introduction, not all readers will want to adopt the Kantian vision of legitimacy. Even if the Kantian political view enjoys some advantages over traditional bioethics theories, the fact of pluralism is not restricted to moral theory; it is also a feature of our political lives, even if we are asking the right questions (that is, even if we are focused on what makes government legitimate, rather than what makes actions moral). What are the implications of the present work for bioethics, that do not depend on readers accepting the Kantian vision of political legitimacy? I think we can draw several important conclusions based on the discussion in this book, relevant to a variety of contexts in bioethics.

At a minimum, it seems that the argument in this book suggests that it should become standard practice in works canvassing theoretical approaches to bioethics (such as introductory bioethics texts or texts on law and bioethics) to distinguish between theories appropriate for determining moral duties and theories appropriate for determining laws and policies. These works already address moral pluralism head on by showing the range of theories developed for answering questions about morality. They should also canvass the plurality of approaches developed for answering questions about politics. They should explain how these theories are designed to address different kinds of questions than are theories of morality. Questions of law and policy are always at least partially questions of secondary rights and duties, and usually raise issues of legitimacy and authority as well. We should not expect theories of primary duties to solve them. Political theories are always relevant and usually necessary in any account about what justifies law or policy. They are thus important not just for questions about how to distribute health care resources justly—currently, approximately the only place where they are usually invoked—but also for any questions about the legal regulation of medicine, such as questions about whether to prohibit organ sales or how much information physicians should be required to give patients. If theory is relevant at all to the normative questions bioethics asks, then it is worth trying to use the right kind of theory.

Much of the bioethics literature is written on a topical basis and seeks to address the ethical aspects of various law and policy issues in health care. There is a rich tradition in this literature of applying various theoretical perspectives to individual issues. This tradition is apparent in the discussion in chapter 3 of the small literature about the implications of Kantian practical philosophy for organs in markets, and in the survey in chapter 8 of the literature attempting to discern the implications of patients' rights for laws governing informed consent. Although most of the articles I discuss in these chapters are either overtly or indirectly Kantian, most of the topical literature in bioethics is not. Even so, we can still draw some conclusions here about how this whole literature could be improved. It should become a standard expectation that articles drawing normative conclusions about law and policy should depend, in part or in whole, on theoretical perspectives capable of sustaining those conclusions. This will usually mean drawing on political rather than moral theories. Moral theories have determinative implications for law and policy only when combined with premises about what makes government just or legitimate or good, as we saw in chapter 2. Without direct attention to general accounts about what governments can or should do, authors drawing political conclusions leave what is arguably the most important premise for drawing such conclusions unexamined. In the case that authors cannot defend recommendations for laws and policies on the basis of a theory of government, they should simply refrain from making those recommendations, or at least acknowledge the nature of the inadequacy in their arguments.

We can also draw a preliminary conclusion about the topical bioethics literature that is focused on moral, rather than legal, issues in the clinical context. Although this literature appears to be far removed from the abstract concerns of political philosophy, in reality it is more closely related than it may appear. There is no way to make normative recommendations that depend in part on the laws that regulate health care, unless we can explain the moral significance of laws and policies. For this we need an account of government authority, and so political philosophy is relevant even here. As we saw in both chapter 6 and chapter 8, laws are sometimes foundational for determining the nature of our moral duties. We may not be able to tell whether an action uses someone else merely as a means unless we know what it means to use a person at all. And for this, we need a background theory of rights and property. Otherwise, the thief can always claim that she does not use her victim as a mere means, she merely uses his stuff. In this vein, we saw further in chapter 8 that abstract moral rights to consent cannot settle the question about what, specifically, is required for consent. For that, we need a political authority that can conclusively settle what is required for valid consent. And so it turns out that the ethical duties of physicians are dependent in part on the laws that stipulate what they must do to get a valid consent. Political philosophy, then, is not relevant merely to questions of law and policy but is also integral to justified conclusions about moral duties in the clinical context as well. Scholarship on clinical ethics will not always need to refer to political theory, but in cases where final recommendations rely to some extent on existing laws and policies, it should.

Finally, we can draw a conclusion that is applicable to the subset of the bioethics literature that does apply Kantian practical philosophy to issues of law and policy. This literature needs to change dramatically. Although it has become the norm, there is no plausible theoretical justification for applying Kant's Categorical Imperative directly to matters of law and policy, or for enforcing Kantian moral duties. Kantian practical philosophy has an important contribution to make to health law and policy, but it is Kant's political, rather than moral, philosophy which is relevant there. Application of Kantian moral philosophy to bioethics dates all the way back to the earliest works in the field—it formed a crucial part of the justification for the principle of respect for persons in the *Belmont Report*,[7] and for the principle of respect for autonomy in early editions of Beauchamp and Childress's *Principles*.[8] Kant's deontological approach has been important in part because it provides a basis for stringent and nonnegotiable duties such as duties to obtain consent, and also because it provides a major alternative to consequentialist visions of ethics. Kant's deontological approach should continue to play an important role in bioethics, but the field needs to reconsider how it applies to law and policy. It is his deontological vision of political legitimacy and authority that are relevant here, and not his discussion of moral duties grounded in the various formulations of the Categorical Imperative. This book provides a vision of how his political philosophy might apply to issues of law and policy, but other Kantian political interpretations are certainly possible. Much work remains to be done to assess the implications of Kantian political philosophy for various issues in bioethics—including, for example, policies regulating the distribution of health care[9] and research on human subjects.

The discovery that bioethics is political should, in the final analysis, be a welcome one. Bioethics has always been political, but it hasn't always been conscious of this fact, and it hasn't developed the tools it needs to deal with questions of law and policy. There is an alternative to either pretending that the field is not political or to simply withdrawing from questions of law and policy. We can develop the tools we need to make normative recommendations for law and policy. We can bring political philosophy into bioethics.

NOTES

1. Arthur Caplan, "'Who Lost China?' a Foreshadowing of Today's Ideological Disputes in Bioethics," *The Hastings Center Report* 35, no. 3 (2005).

2. Leon R. Kass, "Reflections on Public Bioethics: A View from the Trenches," *Kennedy Institute of Ethics Journal* 15, no. 3 (2005).

3. J. D. Moreno, "The End of the Great Bioethics Compromise," *Hastings Center Report* 35, no. 1 (2005).

4. Kass, "Reflections on Public Bioethics: A View from the Trenches."

5. Kass, "Reflections on Public Bioethics: A View from the Trenches."

6. John Evans argues that although bioethicists had long been perceived as representing the values of society, the Bush Council (and especially the backlash to it from liberal bioethicists) revealed publicly that it had mostly represented just one part of the political spectrum. Evans further argues that the Bush Council was an indicator of the "crisis" for the "legitimacy" of public policy bioethics. See John Hyde Evans, *The History and Future of Bioethics: A Sociological View* (New York: Oxford University Press, 2012).

7. H. Tristram Jr. Engelhardt, "Basic Ethical Principles in the Conduct of Biomedical and Behavioral Research Involving Humans Subjects," in *The Belmont Report: Ethical Principles and Guidelines for the Protection of Human Subjects of Research. Appendix Vol. I* (Bethesda, MD: US Department of Health, Education, and Welfare, 1978).

8. Kant's moral philosophy featured in the defense of the principle of respect for autonomy until at least the 5th edition of *Principles*. See Tom L. Beauchamp and James F. Childress, *Principles of Biomedical Ethics*, 5th ed. (New York: Oxford University Press, 2001), 63–64.

9. For an initial attempt at this, see Luke J. Davies, "A Kantian Defense of the Right to Health Care," in *Kantian Theory and Human Rights*, ed. Reidar Maliks and Andreas Follesdal (Routledge, 2013).

Bibliography

Adashi, Eli Y., and I. Glenn Cohen. "An Overdue Executive Order: Reinstating the National Bioethics Commission." *The American Journal of Medicine* (2021).
Alpinar-Şencan, Zümrüt. "Reconsidering Kantian Arguments against Organ Selling." *Medicine, Health Care and Philosophy* 19, no. 1 (2015): 21–31.
Anderson, Scott. "Coercion." In *The Stanford Encyclopedia of Philosophy*, edited by Edward N. Zalta, 2008. http://plato.stanford.edu/archives/fall2008/entries/coercion/.
Annas, George J. *Standard of Care: The Law of American Bioethics.* New York: Oxford University Press, 1993.
Arras, John. "A Taxonomy of Theoretical Work in Bioethics: Supplement to Theory and Bioethics." In *The Stanford Encyclopedia of Philosophy*, edited by Edward N. Zalta, 2020. https://plato.stanford.edu/archives/fall2020/entries/theory-bioethics/supplement.html.
———. "Theory and Bioethics." In *The Stanford Encyclopedia of Philosophy*, edited by Edward N. Zalta, 2020. https://plato.stanford.edu/archives/fall2020/entries/theory-bioethics/.
Arrow, Kenneth. "Uncertainty and the Welfare Economics of Medical Care." *The American Economic Review* 53, no. 5 (1963): 941–73.
Ashcroft, Richard E. "Kant, Mill, Durkheim? Trust and Autonomy in Bioethics and Politics." *Studies in History and Philosophy of Biological and Biomedical Sciences* 34, no. 2 (2003): 359–66.
Association of Bioethics Program Directors, The. "Letter to President Biden." (5/24/21 2021). https://www.bioethicsdirectors.net/wp-content/uploads/2021/06/ABPD-letter-Presidential-Bioethics-Commission.pdf.
Atiyah, Patrick S. *Promises, Morals, and Law.* New York: Oxford University Press, 1981.
Baylis, Francoise. "Persons with Moral Expertise and Moral Experts: Wherein Lies the Difference?" In *Clinical Ethics: Theory and Practice*, edited by C. Barry Hoffmaster, Benjamin Freedman and Gwen Fraser, 89–100. Clifton, N.J.: Humana Press, 1989.
Baylis, Francoise C. "The Health Care Ethics Consultant." *Human Studies* 22, no. 1 (1999): 25–41.

Beauchamp, Tom, and James Childress. "Principles of Biomedical Ethics: Marking Its Fortieth Anniversary." *The American Journal of Bioethics* 19, no. 11 (2019): 9–12.

Beauchamp, Tom L. *Contemporary Issues in Bioethics.* 7th ed. United States: Thomson/Wadsworth, 2008.

———. "The 'Four Principles' Approach to Health Care Ethics." In *Principles of Health Care Ethics*, edited by Richard Edmund Ashcroft, Angus Dawson, Heather Draper and John McMillan, 3–10. New York: Wiley, 2007.

———. "The Origins and Evolution of the Belmont Report." In *Belmont Revisited: Ethical Principles for Research with Human Subjects*, edited by James F. Childress, Eric Mark Meslin and Harold T. Shapiro, 12–25. Washington, DC: Georgetown University Press, 2005.

Beauchamp, Tom L., and James F. Childress. *Principles of Biomedical Ethics.* 8th ed. New York: Oxford University Press, 2019.

———. *Principles of Biomedical Ethics.* 7th ed. New York: Oxford University Press, 2013.

———. *Principles of Biomedical Ethics.* 5th ed. New York: Oxford University Press, 2001.

Bishop, Jeffrey P., and Fabrice Jotterand. "Bioethics as Biopolitics." *The Journal of Medicine and Philosophy* 31, no. 3 (2006): 205–12.

Bole III, Thomas J. "The Sale of Organs and Obligations to One's Body: Inferences from the History of Ethics." In *Persons and Their Bodies*, edited by Mark J. Cherry, 331–50. Boston: Kluwer Academic, 1999.

Brody, Baruch A. "Limiting Life-Prolonging Medical Treatment: A Comparative Analysis of the President's Commission and the New York State Task Force." In *Society's Choices Social and Ethical Decision Making in Biomedicine*, edited by Ruth Ellen. Bulger, Elizabeth Meyer. Bobby, Harvey V. Fineberg, 307–34. Washington, D.C.: National Academy Press, 1995.

Brummett, Abram, and Christopher J Ostertag. "Two Troubling Trends in the Conversation over Whether Clinical Ethics Consultants Have Ethics Expertise." *HEC Forum* 30, no. 2 (2017): 157–69.

Buchanan, Allen. "Political Legitimacy and Democracy." *Ethics* 112, no. 4 (2002): 689–719.

Byrd, B. Sharon, and Joachim Hruschka. *Kant's Doctrine of Right: A Commentary.* New York: Cambridge University Press, 2010.

Callahan, Daniel. *Abortion: Law, Choice and Morality*. New York: Macmillan, 1970.

Campbell, Alastair V. *Bioethics: The Basics.* Milton Park, Abingdon, Oxon: Routledge, 2013.

Caplan, Arthur. "'Who Lost China?' a Foreshadowing of Today's Ideological Disputes in Bioethics." *The Hastings Center Report* 35, no. 3 (2005): 12–13.

Carlson, Robert V., Kenneth M. Boyd, and David J. Webb. "The Revision of the Declaration of Helsinki: Past, Present and Future." *British Journal of Clinical Pharmacology* 57, no. 6 (2004): 695–713.

Casarett, David J., Frona Daskal, and John Lantos. "The Authority of the Clinical Ethicist." *Hastings Center Report* 28, no. 6 (1998): 6.

Chadwick, Ruth. "The Market for Bodily Parts: Kant and Duties to Oneself." *Journal of Applied Philosophy* 6, no. 2 (1989): 129–40.

Charo, R. Alta. "The Hunting of the Snark: The Moral Status of Embryos, Right-to-Lifers, and Third World Women." *Stanford Law & Policy Review* 6, no. 2 (1995): 11–37.

Chon, W. J., M. A. Josephson, E. J. Gordon, Y. T. Becker, P. Witkowski, D. J. Arwindekar, A. Naik, et al. "When the Living and the Deceased Cannot Agree on Organ Donation: A Survey of Us Organ Procurement Organizations (OPOS)." *American Journal of Transplantation*, 14, no. 1 (2014): 172–77.

Cohen, Barbara. "Surrogate Mothers: Whose Baby Is It?". *American Journal of Law & Medicine* 10, no. 3 (1984): 243–85.

Cohen, Cynthia B. "Public Policy and the Sale of Human Organs." *Kennedy Institute of Ethics Journal* 12, no. 1 (2002): 47–64.

Cohen, Cynthia B. "Selling Bits and Pieces of Humans to Make Babies: The Gift of the Magi Revisited." *The Journal of Medicine and Philosophy* 24, no. 3 (1999): 288–306.

Curran, Charles E. *Politics, Medicine, and Christian Ethics: A Dialogue with Paul Ramsey*. Philadelphia: Fortress Press, 1973.

Daniels, Norman. *Just Health Care*. New York: Cambridge University Press, 1985.

———. *Just Health: Meeting Health Needs Fairly*. New York: Cambridge University Press, 2008.

Davies, Luke J. "A Kantian Defense of the Right to Health Care." In *Kantian Theory and Human Rights*, edited by Reidar Maliks and Andreas Follesdal, 70–88: Routledge, 2013.

———. "Kant on Welfare: Five Unsuccessful Defences." *Kantian Review* 25, no. 1 (2020): 1–25.

Dawson, Angus. "Editorial: Political Philosophy and Public Health Ethics." *Public Health Ethics* 2, no. 2 (2009): 121.

DeGrazia, David, Thomas A. Mappes, and Jeffrey Brand-Ballard. *Biomedical Ethics*. New York: McGraw-Hill Higher Education, 2011.

Department of Health, Education, and Welfare. "45 CFR 46. Protection of Human Subjects." *Federal Register* 39, no. 105 (1974): 18914–20.

Dolgin, Janet L., and Lois L. Shepherd. *Bioethics and the Law*. New York: Aspen Publishers, 2009.

Dranseika, Vilius, Jan Piasecki, and Marcin Waligora. "Relevant Information and Informed Consent in Research: In Defense of the Subjective Standard of Disclosure." *Science and Engineering Ethics* 23, no. 1 (2016): 215–25.

Emanuel, Ezekiel J. *The Ends of Human Life: Medical Ethics in a Liberal Polity*. Cambridge, MA: Harvard University Press, 1991.

Emanuel, Ezekiel J., and Linda L. Emanuel. "Four Models of the Physician-Patient Relationship." In *Ethical Issues in Modern Medicine*, edited by Bonnie Steinbock, John Arras and Alex John London, 67–76. Boston: McGraw-Hill, 2003.

Engelhardt, H. T. "The Injustice of Enforced Equal Access to Transplant Operations: Rethinking Reckless Claims of Fairness." *The Journal of Law, Medicine, & Ethics* 35, no. 2 (2007): 256–64.

Engelhardt, H. Tristram. *The Foundations of Bioethics*. New York: Oxford University Press, 1996.

———. "Why Clinical Bioethics So Rarely Gives Morally Normative Guidance." In *Bioethics Critically Reconsidered: Having Second Thoughts*, edited by H. Tristram Engelhardt, 151–74. Dordrecht: Springer, 2012.

Engelhardt, H. Tristram Jr. "Basic Ethical Principles in the Conduct of Biomedical and Behavioral Research Involving Humans Subjects." In *The Belmont Report: Ethical Principles and Guidelines for the Protection of Human Subjects of Research. Appendix Vol. I*. Bethesda, MD: US Department of Health, Education, and Welfare, 1978.

Engelhardt Jr., H. Tristram. "The Body for Fun, Beneficence and Profit: A Variation on a Post-Modern Theme." In *Persons and Their Bodies: Rights, Responsibilities, Relationships*, edited by Mark J. Cherry, 277–301. Dordrecht; Boston: Kluwer Academic, 1999.

Evans, John Hyde. *The History and Future of Bioethics: A Sociological View*. New York: Oxford University Press, 2012.

———. *Playing God? Human Genetic Engineering and the Rationalization of Public Bioethical Debate*. Chicago: University of Chicago Press, 2002.

Fabre, Cècile. *Whose Body Is It Anyway? Justice and the Integrity of the Person*. Oxford: Clarendon Press, 2009.

Faden, Ruth R., and Tom L. Beauchamp. *A History and Theory of Informed Consent*. New York: Oxford University Press, 1986.

Flikschuh, Katrin. "Innate Right and Acquired Right in Arthur Ripstein's Force and Freedom." *Jurisprudence* 1, no. 2 (2010): 295–304.

———. *Kant and Modern Political Philosophy*. New York: Cambridge University Press, 2000.

Flynn, Jennifer. "Theory and Bioethics." In *The Stanford Encyclopedia of Philosophy*, edited by Edward N. Zalta, 2021. https://plato.stanford.edu/archives/spr2021/entries/theory-bioethics/.

Fried, Charles. *Contract as Promise: A Theory of Contractual Obligation*. Cambridge, Mass.: Harvard University Press, 1981.

Furrow, Barry R., Thomas L. Greaney, Sandra H. Johnson, Timothy S. Jost, Robert L. Schwartz, Brietta R. Clark, Erin C. Fuse Brown, Robert Gatter, and Elizabeth Pendo. *Bioethics: Health Care Law and Ethics*. 8th ed. St. Paul, MN: West Academic Publishing, 2018.

Garrison, Marsha, and Carl Schneider. *The Law of Bioethics: Individual Autonomy and Social Regulation*. 2nd ed. St. Paul, MN: Thomson/West, 2009.

Gerrand, Nicole. "The Misuse of Kant in the Debate About a Market for Human Body Parts." *Journal of Applied Philosophy* 16, no. 1 (1999): 59–67.

Gert, Bernard, Charles M. Culver, and K. Danner Clouser. *Bioethics: A Systematic Approach*. 2nd ed. New York: Oxford University Press, 2006.

Ghods, Ahad J., and Shekoufeh Savaj. "Iranian Model of Paid and Regulated Living-Unrelated Kidney Donation." *Clinical Journal of the American Society of Nephrology* 1, no. 6 (2006): 1136–45.

Gill, Michael B., and Robert M. Sade. "Paying for Kidneys: The Case against Prohibition." *Kennedy Institute of Ethics Journal* 12, no. 1 (2002): 17–45.
Glantz, Leonard H., George J. Annas, Michael A. Grodin, and Wendy K. Mariner. "Research in Developing Countries: Taking Benefit Seriously." In *Ethical Issues in Modern Medicine*, edited by Bonnie Steinbock, John Arras and Alex John London, 781–86. Boston: McGraw-Hill, 2003.
Glazier, Alexandra K. "Organ Donation and the Principles of Gift Law." *Clinical Journal of the American Society of Nephrology* 13, no. 8 (2018): 1283–84.
Gray, Bradford H. "Bioethics Commissions: What Can We Learn from Past Successes and Failures?". In *Society's Choices: Social and Ethical Decision Making in Biomedicine*, edited by Ruth Ellen. Bulger, Elizabeth Meyer. Bobby and Harvey V. Fineberg, 261–306. Washington, D.C.: National Academy Press, 1995.
Green, Ronald M. "What Does It Mean to Use Someone as 'a Means Only': Rereading Kant." *Kennedy Institute of Ethics Journal* 11, no. 3 (2001): 247–61.
Gregor, Mary. "Kant on Welfare Legislation." *Logos* 6 (1985): 49–59.
———. "Translator's Note on the Text of the Metaphysics of Morals." Edited and Translated by Mary J. Gregor. In *Practical Philosophy*. The Cambridge Edition of the Works of Immanuel Kant, 355–59. New York: Cambridge University Press, 1996.
Harré, Rom. "Bodily Obligations." *Cogito* 1, no. 3 (1987): 15–19.
Heubel, Friedrich, and Nicola Biller-Andorno. "The Contribution of Kantian Moral Theory to Contemporary Medical Ethics: A Critical Analysis." *Medicine, Health Care and Philosophy* 8, no. 1 (2005): 5–18.
Hodgson, Louis Philippe. "Kant on the Right to Freedom: A Defense." *Ethics* 120, no. 4 (2010): 791–819.
Hohfeld, Wesley Newcomb. *Fundamental Legal Conceptions*. Edited by W. Cook. New Haven: Yale University Press, 1919.
Holm, Søren. "Bioethics Down Under—Medical Ethics Engages with Political Philosophy." *Journal of Medical Ethics* 31, no. 1 (2005): 1.
Huemer, Michael. The Problem of Political Authority: An Examination of the Right to Coerce and the Duty to Obey. New York: Palgrave Macmillan, 2013.
Iltis, Ana S, and Mark Sheehan. "Expertise, Ethics Expertise, and Clinical Ethics Consultation: Achieving Terminological Clarity." *The Journal of Medicine and Philosophy* 41, no. 4 (2016): 416–33.
Jonsen, Albert R. "A History of Bioethics as Discipline and Discourse." In *Bioethics: An Introduction to the History, Methods, and Practice*, edited by N. A. S. Jecker, A. R. Jonsen and R. A. Pearlman, 3–16: Jones and Bartlett Publishers, 2007.
Jonsen, Albert R. *The Birth of Bioethics*. New York: Oxford University Press, 1998.
Kant, Immanuel. "The Doctrine of Right." Edited and Translated by Mary J. Gregor. In *The Metaphysics of Morals*, 1–138. New York: Cambridge University Press, 1996.
———. "Groundwork of the Metaphysics of Morals." Edited and Translated by Mary J. Gregor. In *Practical Philosophy*. The Cambridge Edition of the Works of Immanuel Kant, 37–108. New York: Cambridge University Press, 1996.

———. *Lectures on Ethics.* Translated by Louis Infield. Indianapolis: Hackett Pub. Co., 1980.

———. *Lectures on Ethics.* New York: Cambridge University Press, 1997.

———. "On a Supposed Right to Lie from Philanthropy." Edited and Translated by Mary J. Gregor. In *Practical Philosophy.* The Cambridge Edition of the Works of Immanuel Kant, 605–15. New York: Cambridge University Press, 1996.

———. "Review of Hufeland's Essay on the Principle of Natural Right." Edited and Translated by Mary J. Gregor. In *Practical Philosophy.* The Cambridge Edition of the Works of Immanuel Kant, 109–17. New York: Cambridge University Press, 1996.

Kass, Leon. *Life, Liberty, and the Defense of Dignity: The Challenge for Bioethics.* 1st ed. San Francisco: Encounter Books, 2002.

Kass, Leon R. "Organs for Sale? Propriety, Property, and the Price of Progress." *The Public Interest*, no. 107 (1993): 65–86.

Kass, Leon R. "Reflections on Public Bioethics: A View from the Trenches." *Kennedy Institute of Ethics Journal* 15, no. 3 (2005): 221–50.

Kaufman, Alexander. *Welfare in the Kantian State.* New York: Oxford University Press, 1999.

Kerstein, Samuel. "Autonomy, Moral Constraints, and Markets in Kidneys." *Journal of Medicine and Philosophy* 34, no. 6 (2009): 573–85.

———. "Kantian Condemnation of Commerce in Organs." *Kennedy Institute of Ethics Journal* 19, no. 2 (2009): 147–69.

Ketchum, Sara Ann. "Selling Babies and Selling Bodies." *Hypatia* 4, no. 3 (1989): 116–27.

Korsgaard, Christine. "The Right to Lie: Kant on Dealing with Evil." *Philosophy and Public Affairs* 15, no. 4 (1986): 325–49.

Kristinsson, Sigurdur. "Autonomy and Informed Consent: A Mistaken Association?" *Medicine, Health Care and Philosophy* 10, no. 3 (2007): 253–64.

Kymlicka, Will. "Moral Philosophy and Public Policy: The Case of New Reproductive Technologies." In *Philosophical Perspectives on Bioethics*, edited by L W Sumner and Joseph M Boyle, 244–70. Toronto: University of Toronto Press, 1996.

LaFrance, Arthur B. *Bioethics: Health Care, Human Rights, and the Law.* 2nd ed. 1 vols. Newark, NJ: Matthew Bender, 2006.

Lowi, Theodore J. "Law Vs. Public Policy: A Critical Exploration." *Cornell Journal of Law and Public Policy* 12, no. 3 (2003): 493–501.

MacDougall, D. Robert. "Intervention Principles in Pediatric Health Care: The Difference between Physicians and the State." *Theoretical Medicine and Bioethics* 40, no. 4 (2019): 279–97.

———. "Liberalism, Authority, and Bioethics Commissions." *Theoretical Medicine and Bioethics* 34, no. 6 (2013): 461–77.

———. "Sometimes Merely as a Means: Why Kantian Philosophy Requires the Legalization of Kidney Sales." *The Journal of Medicine and Philosophy* 44, no. 3 (2019): 314–34.

Manson, Neil C., and Onora O'Neill. *Rethinking Informed Consent in Bioethics.* Cambridge: Cambridge University Press, 2007.

McDougall, Rosalind. "Systematic Reviews in Bioethics: Types, Challenges, and Value." *The Journal of Medicine and Philosophy* 39, no. 1 (2014): 89–97.

Menikoff, Jerry. *Law and Bioethics: An Introduction*. Washington, D.C.: Georgetown University Press, 2001.

Merle, Jean-Christophe. "A Kantian Argument for a Duty to Donate One's Own Organs. A Reply to Nicole Gerrand." *Journal of Applied Philosophy* 17, no. 1 (2000): 93–101.

Mill, John Stuart. *On Liberty*. New York: Liberal Arts Press, 1956.

Miller, Franklin G, and Alan Wertheimer. "Preface to a Theory of Consent Transactions: Beyond Valid Consent." In *The Ethics of Consent: Theory and Practice*, edited by Franklin G. Miller and Alan Wertheimer, 79–105. Oxford: Oxford University Press, 2010.

Miller, Franklin G., and Alan Wertheimer. "The Fair Transaction Model of Informed Consent: An Alternative to Autonomous Authorization." *Kennedy Institute of Ethics Journal* 21, no. 3 (2011): 201–18.

Morelli, Mario. "Commerce in Organs: A Kantian Critique." *Journal of Social Philosophy* 30, no. 2 (2004): 315–24.

Moreno, J. D. "The End of the Great Bioethics Compromise." *Hastings Center Report* 35, no. 1 (2005): 14–15.

Munson, Ronald. *Intervention and Reflection: Basic Issues in Bioethics*. 8th ed. Boston, MA: Wadsworth, Cengage Learning, 2008.

Munzer, Stephen R. "Kant and Property Rights in Body Parts." *Canadian Journal of Law and Jurisprudence* 6 (1993): 319.

———. "An Uneasy Case against Property Rights in Body Parts." *Social Philosophy and Policy* 11, no. 2 (1994): 259–86.

Narveson, Jan. *You and the State: A Fairly Brief Introduction to Political Philosophy*. Lanham: Rowman & Littlefield Publishers, 2008.

National Conference of Commissioners on Uniform State Laws. "Uniform Determination of Death Act." 1980.

Nozick, Robert. *Anarchy, State, and Utopia*. New York: Basic Books, 1974.

———. "Coercion." In *Philosophy, Science, and Method: Essays in Honor of Ernest Nagel*, edited by Sidney Morgenbesser, Patrick Suppes and Morton Gabriel White, 440–72. New York: St. Martin's Press, 1969.

O'Neill, Onora. *Autonomy and Trust in Bioethics*. Cambridge: Cambridge University Press, 2003.

———. "Kant and the Social Contract Tradition." In *Kant Actuel: Hommage À Pierre Laberge*, edited by François Duchesneau, Claude Piché and Guy Lafrance, 185–200. Montréal: Bellarmin, 2000.

Outka, G. "Social Justice and Equal Access to Health Care." *The Journal of Religious Ethics* 2, no. 1 (1974): 11–32.

Pallikkathayil, Japa. "Deriving Morality from Politics: Rethinking the Formula of Humanity." *Ethics* 121, no. 1 (2010): 116–47.

———. "Persons and Bodies." In *Freedom and Force: Essays on Kant's Legal Philosophy*, edited by Sari Kisilevsky and Martin Jay Stone. Portland: Hart Publishing, 2017.

Pereboom, Derk. "Kant's Transcendental Arguments." In *The Stanford Encyclopedia of Philosophy*, edited by Edward N. Zalta, 2019. https://plato.stanford.edu/archives/spr2019/entries/kant-transcendental/.

Pogge, Thomas W. "Is Kant's Rechtslehre Comprehensive?" *The Southern Journal of Philosophy* 36, no. S1 (1998): 161–87.

Potter, Van Rensselaer. "Bioethics, the Science of Survival." *Perspectives in Biology and Medicine* 14, no. 1 (1970): 127–53.

Powers, Thomas M. "The Integrity of Body: Kantian Moral Constraints on the Physical Self." In *Persons and Their Bodies: Rights, Responsibilities, Relationships*, edited by Mark J. Cherry, 209–32. Boston: Kluwer Academic, 1999.

President's Commission for the Study of Ethical Problems in Medicine and Biomedical and Behavioral Research. *Deciding to Forego Life-Sustaining Treatment: A Report on the Ethical, Medical, and Legal Issues in Treatment Decisions*. Washington, DC: U.S. G.P.O., 1983.

———. Defining Death: A Report on the Medical, Legal and Ethical Issues in the Determination of Death. Washington, D.C.: U.S. G.P.O., 1981.

Rachels, James. "Active and Passive Euthanasia." *The New England Journal of Medicine* 292, no. 2 (1975): 78–80.

Rasmussen, Lisa M. "Clinical Ethics Consultants Are Not "Ethics" Experts—but They Do Have Expertise." *The Journal of Medicine and Philosophy* 41, no. 4 (2016): 384–400.

Rawls, John. *Political Liberalism*. New York: Columbia Univ. Press, 2005.

———. *A Theory of Justice*. Cambridge, Massachusetts: Belknap Press of Harvard University Press, 1971.

Reich, W. T. "The Word 'Bioethics': Its Birth and the Legacies of Those Who Shaped It." *Kennedy Institute of Ethics Journal* 4, no. 4 (1994): 319–35.

Reich, Warren Thomas. "The Word 'Bioethics': The Struggle over Its Earliest Meanings." *Kennedy Institute of Ethics Journal* 5, no. 1 (1995): 19–34.

Ripstein, Arthur. *Force and Freedom: Kant's Legal and Political Philosophy*. Cambridge, Mass.: Harvard University Press, 2009.

Rousseau, Jean-Jacques. *A Discourse Upon the Origin and the Foundation of Inequality among Mankind*. New York: Bartleby.com, 2001. http://bartleby.com/34/3/.

Schaller, Barry R. *Understanding Bioethics and the Law: The Promises and Perils of the Brave New World of Biotechnology*. Westport, Conn.: Praeger, 2008.

Seel, Gerhard. "How Does Kant Justify the Universal Objective Validity of the Law of Right?". *International Journal of Philosophical Studies* 17, no. 1 (2009): 71–94.

Shell, Susan M. "Kant's Concept of Human Dignity." In *Human Dignity and Bioethics*, edited by Edmund D. Pellegrino, Adam Schulman, Thomas W. Merrill and The President's Council on Bioethics, 333–49. Notre Dame, Ind.: University of Notre Dame Press, 2009.

Sherwin, Susan. *No Longer Patient: Feminist Ethics and Health Care*. Philadelphia: Temple University Press, 1992.

Sherwin, Susan B., and F. Baylis. "The Feminist Health Care Ethics Consultant as Architect and Advocate." *Public Affairs Quarterly* 17, no. 2 (2003): 141–58.

Simmons, A. John. *Political Philosophy.* New York: Oxford University Press, 2008.
Sokol, Daniel K. "Update on the UK Law on Consent." *British Medical Journal* 350 (2015): h1481.
Spielman, Bethany. *Bioethics in Law.* Totowa, N.J.: Humana Press, 2007.
Steinbock, Bonnie, John Arras, and Alex John London. *Ethical Issues in Modern Medicine.* 6th ed. Boston: McGraw-Hill, 2003.
Stempsey, William E. "Organ Markets and Human Dignity: On Selling Your Body and Soul." *Christian Bioethics* 6, no. 2 (2000): 195–204.
Studdert, David M., Michelle M. Mello, Marin K. Levy, Russell L. Gruen, Edward J. Dunn, E. John Orav, and Troyen A. Brennan. "Geographic Variation in Informed Consent Law: Two Standards for Disclosure of Treatment Risks." *Journal of Empirical Legal Studies* 4, no. 1 (2007): 103–24.
Taylor, James Stacey. "Autonomy and Informed Consent: A Much Misunderstood Relationship." *The Journal of Value Inquiry* 38, no. 3 (2005): 383–91.
———. *Stakes and Kidneys: Why Markets in Human Body Parts Are Morally Imperative.* Burlington, VT: Ashgate Pub., 2005.
Taylor, R. S. "Self-Ownership and Transplantable Human Organs." *Public Affairs Quarterly* (2007).
Taylor, Robert S. "A Kantian Defense of Self-Ownership." *Journal of Political Philosophy* 12, no. 1 (2004): 65–78.
———. "Self-Ownership and Transplantable Human Organs." *Public Affairs Quarterly* 21, no. 1 (2007): 89–107.
Tong, Rosemarie. *Feminist Approaches to Bioethics: Theoretical Reflections and Practical Applications.* Boulder, Colo.: Westview Press, 1997.
Toulmin, Stephen. "The Tyranny of Principles." *The Hastings Center Report* 11, no. 6 (1981): 31–39.
Uleman, Jennifer K. "External Freedom in Kant's 'Rechtslehre': Political, Metaphysical." *Philosophy and Phenomenological Research* 68, no. 3 (2004): 578–601.
Vaughn, Lewis. *Bioethics: Principles, Issues, and Cases.* 3rd ed. New York: Oxford University Press, 2017.
Veitch, Kenneth. *The Jurisdiction of Medical Law.* Burlington, VT: Ashgate, 2007.
Wenar, Leif. "Rights." In *The Stanford Encyclopedia of Philosophy*, edited by Edward N. Zalta, 2010. http://plato.stanford.edu/archives/fall2010/entries/rights/.
Wilkinson, Dominic J. C. "Selling Organs and Souls: Should the State Prohibit 'Demeaning' Practices?" *Journal of Bioethical Inquiry* 1, no. 1 (2004): 27–31.
Willaschek, Marcus. "Why the Doctrine of Right Does Not Belong in the Metaphysics of Morals." *Annual Review of Law and Ethics* 5 (1997): 205–27.
Wolff, Robert Paul. *In Defense of Anarchism.* New York: Harper & Row, 1970.
Wood, Allen. "Right and Ethics: Arthur Ripstein's Force and Freedom." In *Freedom and Force: Essays on Kant's Legal Philosophy*, edited by Sari Kisilevsky and Martin Jay Stone, 143–64. Portland, OR: Hart Publishing, 2017.
Wood, Allen W. "The Final Form of Kant's Practical Philosophy." *Southern Journal of Philosophy* 36 (1997): 1–20.

———. "The Supreme Principle of Morality." In *The Cambridge Companion to Kant and Modern Philosophy*, edited by Paul Guyer, 342–80. New York: Cambridge University Press, 2006.

Index

abortion, 27
acquired right, 131–37, 164–65
action, 94, 111–12, 145–54, 178–79, 187
assurance, 135–36, 139–40
attributes of a citizen, 207n27
authority of the state, 6–7, 10, 51–52, 140–42, 156n26, 165–66, 168, 197–98; *See also* legitimacy, political; to obey *under* duty(duties)
autonomy: Kantian, 72, 78, 92, 163, 188; and obedience to the law, 102n11; principle of respect for, 39, 40, 163, 187–88, 193, 202, 215n8; rights, 187–88; *See also* Formula of Autonomy *under* Categorical Imperative

beneficence, principle of, 39, 51, 58n29, 68
Belmont Commission, 19, 21–23, 37–38, 209–10, 214
Belmont Report, 15, 19, 37–38; principles of, 19, 22–23, 37, 209
bioethicists: clinical, 25, 33n43; conservative, 209–10; contribution to law and policy, 14–15, 186–87; giving policy advice, 17–23, 205–6, 212–13; liberal, 209–10, 215n6
bioethics: clinical, 3, 17, 25–27, 29, 33n43, 206, 213–14; discipline of, 17, 18, 31n13; history of, 18–23, 36–39, 209–11; introductions to, 212; Kantian, 3, 214; methodological problems, 1–3, 205–6, 211; philosophical methods in, 1–2; qualitative empirical reviews in, 2, 10n2; subject matter of, 23–25; and theory, 7, 35; theories of, 39–52, 209–11; tools of, 1–2, 17, 35, 205, 214; *See also* political philosophy; principles
body (bodies), 73–75, 130–31, 176–77, 182n6, 184n43; property in, 78, 83n36; rights to, 164–65, 183n40; *See also* kidney(s), person(s)

Categorical Imperative, 5, 64–66, 68, 72–73, 78–79, 80–81, 87–88, 91–93, 95–97, 100–1, 120, 127n35, 144–45, 203, 214; *See also* Formula of Autonomy; Formula of Humanity; Formula of Universal Law; human dignity
children, 155n6

227

choice, 107, 109, 110, 125n6, 125n10, 131, 132, 162; *See also* of choice *under* freedom; united choice

civil condition, 127n26, 136–38, 138–43, 157n42, 158n47; duty to establish, 137–42, 156n23, 157n42; right to establish, 137–38; as solution to the problem of violence, 197–98; *See also* public right; state, the; state of nature

coercion, 5, 93, 135, 179–80, 188–89; as an activity of governments, 88; to adopt ends, 93; in bioethics, 126n24; in contrast to other forms of influence, 95; credible and severe threat account, 117–20, 153–54; and Formula of Humanity, 97–98, 144–54; and Formula of Universal Law, 96–98; hindrance to freedom account, 112–13, 117–20; in medicine, 127n33; moral, 120–23, 127n35, 144–45, 157n38, 157n48; morally justifiable, 144–54; motivation for, 120–22; reciprocal, 114–15, 139, 151; rightful, 113–15, 120–25, 138; as a use or threat of force, 96, 112; *See also* assurance; security, unequal

commissions, government, 7, 14–15, 19–23, 55; Human Gene Therapy Subcommittee of the Recombinant DNA Advisory Commission, 22–23; National Commission for the Protection of Human Subjects of Biomedical and Behavioral Research. *See* Belmont Commission; President's Commission for the Study of Ethical Problems in Medicine and Biomedical and Behavioral Research, 20–21; Presidential Council on Bioethics, 209–10, 215n6

common morality, 39–40, 48–9, 57–58n14, 209–11

Common Rule, 19–20, 38

comprehensive doctrines, 71–72

condition, rightful, 111, 138, 151

consensus, 210–11

consent, 6–7, 50, 73, 99, 109, 124, 131, 162–63, 170–72, 176, 178–80, 182n4, 185–86, 194–98; actual, 138–39, 141, 156n28, 158n43; to being used, 149–52; to coercion, 96–97, 103n24, 153–54; hypothetical, 141, 156n28; modal, 156n28; to the original contract, 138–39, 140–41; to the rights of others in the civil condition, 157–58n42; tacit, 158n43; *See also* contract(s); informed consent; legitimate *under* law(s); united choice; united will of all; volenti rule

contract(s), 120, 169, 189; breach of, 169, 171; original, 138–39, 156n20; as sign of consent, 176, 180; unenforceable, 126n18, 174–77, 179–81

contradiction in conception, 97, 103n25; in practical reason, 64–66, 157n42; in the will, 103n25

dead donor rule, 15

death, definition of, 15

deception, 65–66, 96–97, 104n28, 146–48, 188–89

Deciding to Forego Life-Sustaining Treatment, 14, 20–21

delivery, 170–72, 180; *See also* contract(s); promise

democracy, 99, 141, 143, 156n27

Defining Death, 15, 21

disclose, physician's duty to. *See* to inform *under* duty

dismemberment, 75, 84n45, 172; *See also* self–mutilation

division, fallacy of, 73–75, 83–84n43, 174

drug innovator, case of, 146–48

duty (duties): to coerce, 184n48; contrast with rights, 108; division of, 157n45, 183n27; of government, 9; imperfect, 152, 158n45; to inform, 7, 25, 185–93, 197–98, 200, 203–5; Kantian moral, 64–66, 188, 203–5; to obey the law, 26, 27–29, 30, 122, 140–41, 153, 156n26, 203–5, 208n34; perfect, 158n45, 173–74, 183n30, 183n33; of physicians, 36, 46–47, 203–5, 213; primary moral, 9, 41, 47, 48, 55–56, 78–81, 85n68, 89, 188, 208n34, 212; secondary moral, 41–42, 57n19, 78, 89–90, 211–12; *See also* duty to establish *under* civil condition; ends that are also duties; internal duties of right; Universal Principle of Right

ends that are also duties, 94–95, 157n34
equality: 98–100, 124–25, 134–36, 143–44, 201–2
euthanasia, 14, 24, 32–3n39, 178

Formula of Autonomy, 65, 92
Formula of Humanity, 6, 65, 67–68, 72, 79, 89, 93, 97–99, 104n28, 120, 145–54, 157nn37–38, 157n42, 158–59n48, 203–5; *See also* and Formula of Humanity *under* coercion
Formula of Universal Law, 65, 93, 96–97, 99, 103n24, 104n28, 157n37; *See also* Formula of Universal Law *under* coercion
freedom: of choice, 75, 84n45, 108–10; created by universal law, 110; equal, 195–98, 200–1; external, 109, 126n13, 166–68; under universal law, 115; *See also* free *under* persons; hindrance to freedom account *under* coercion

government: activities, special, 79, 88–89; defined and distinguished from the state, 33n46; monopoly on political activities, 88–89, 98–100, 124, 138, 143–44; premises about, 4, 27–30; republican, 156n27; as subject of political philosophy, 29; *See also* authority of the state; democracy; duty; legitimacy, political

happiness, 142–43, 152, 157n34
harm, 119–20, 153
The Hastings Center, 18, 19
health law and policy: as government activities, 27–29, 89–90; ideal normative justification of, 27–29; methods of justification, 1–2; moral philosophy approach to justifying, 5, 6; moral status of, 26; *See also* law(s)
human dignity, 68–70, 71–73, 77, 78–79, 82n28, 83n43, 89, 90, 94, 99
human genetic engineering, 22
humanity, 43, 97, 130–31
hypothetical imperative, 64, 156–57n32

idea of reason, 156n22
incentive, 92, 94
indeterminacy, problem of, 195–97
information asymmetries, 190, 192–93, 207n23
informed consent, 25, 72, 163, 185–93; bioethics accounts of, 187–91; in research, 206n5; waivers of, 204, 208n32; *See also* consent; to inform *under* duty (duties); standards for informed consent, legal
innate right, 126n18, 154, 155n3, 155n6, 157n42, 165, 168, 175; and bodies, 130–31, 182n6; and consent, 194–95; and contracts for kidneys, 180; defined, 130; and the duty to enter a civil condition, 138, 141, 143, 144; and internal duties of right, 172–73, 175; and laws in a civil condition, 197–98; priority

230 *Index*

over acquired right, 164; and the subjective standard, 200–1; *See also* acquired right
Institutional Review Board, 20
interests, 165, 167–68, 193
internal duties of right, 172–80, 183nn27–8;
intuitions, 106

justice: distributive, 44–46, 53, 107, 142–43, 166–68, 212; health, 55; Kant's theory of, 100–1; non-distributive aspects of, 44–45; and oppression, 49–50; principle of, 39, 44–46

Kant's moral philosophy. *See* Categorical Imperative; Kantian *under* theory; relationship to Kant's moral philosophy, *under* Kant's political philosophy
Kant's political philosophy: importance for bioethics, 2–3, 205–6, 211–12, 214; relationship to Kant's moral philosophy, 5, 9, 10n1, 101, 104n31, 127n35, 154, 174, 183n34
Kennedy Institute of Ethics, 19
kidneys: as constitutive parts of persons, 176–77; as property, 75, 78, 180, 184n49; *See also* body (bodies)
kidney markets. *See* kidney sales
kidney donation, 68, 69, 84n56, 76–78, 178–80; *See also* organ donation
kidney sales, 6, 15, 76, 161; contracts for, 170–72, 174–76; legal prohibitions against, 4–6, 31n10, 68, 70, 71, 73, 77, 165–68, 178–81; morality of, 174, 176–77; and the poor, 166–68; right to, 164, 167–68; *See also* kidney donations; kidney purchases; organ sales; unenforceable *under* contract(s)
kidney purchases, 165–66

killing and letting die, distinction between, 14, 32n39, 59n35

law(s): defined and distinguished from policy, 30n2; enforcement of, 16, 27, 30n2, 88–90, 95, 99–100, 118, 127n33, 145, 153–54; legitimate, 140–43, 153, 168, 181, 197–202; universal, 99, 110, 111–12, 113–15, 119, 123, 124, 130, 132, 134, 139, 196–98; *See also* contract(s); enforcing *under* morality; health law and policy; legal prohibitions against *under* kidney sales; standards for informed consent, legal
legitimacy, political, 10, 29, 211; challenges from Kantian theory, 90–101; defined, 89; distinguished from authority, 141, 156n26; limits of, 141–42; problem of, 5, 78–79, 88–90; solution to problem of, 115–25, 143–44; theories of, 3, 181, 205–6; *See also* authority of the state; legitimate *under* law(s)
living will, 13, 15
lying. *See* deception

masturbation, 71, 177, 180, 183n33
metaphysics, Kantian, 73–75; *See also* body (bodies), person(s)
monopoly. *See* monopoly on political activities *under* government
moral epistemology, 51
moral philosophy, 2–3, 5–6, 10n1; *See also* theory
morality: enforcing, 6, 43, 51, 80, 85n68, 91–94, 123–24, 167, 210–11; relationship to the law, 7, 9, 27–29, 43–44, 53, 144–54, 203–6, 213–14; *See also* common morality
mutilation: consensual, 178–80; self-, 66, 75–77, 84n49, 174, 178; *See also* dismemberment

National Organ Transplantation Act, 15

non-maleficence, principle of, 39, 46

obligation, unilateral imposition of: problem of, 134, 136–37, 139, 195; solved by the civil condition, 137–38, 139, 144; *See also* indeterminacy, problem of
organ donation, 15, 174; *See also* kidney donation
organ markets. *See* organ sales
Organ Procurement and Transplantation Network, 15
organ sales, 6, 15, 161, 181; Critics of Kantian arguments for prohibitions of, 71–80; Kant's views on moral permissibility of, 66, 77–78, 83n36; Kantian arguments for legal prohibitions of, 67–70; political philosophy in debate about Kant and, 78–80; *See also* kidney sales
organ transplant, 13–14

parents, 155n6
paternalism, 78–79, 167–68, 193
permission, principle of, 50–52
person(s), 73, 126n6, 131, 164, 168, 176–77; free, 125–26n10, 155n6; mentally disabled, 155n6; status as right–holders, 173–74; things, distinguished from, 73, 173–74; *See also* body (bodies); metaphysics, Kantian
physician-assisted suicide, 24, 26, 27–29, 32–33n39, 46–47, 208n33; *See also* euthanasia, suicide
pluralism, 8, 20, 36–39, 47–48, 50, 209–12; *See also* and pluralism *under* principlism
polarization, 210
policy. *See* defined and distinguished from policy *under* law
political obligation. *See* to obey *under* duty(duties)
political philosophy: absence in bioethics, 2–4, 17, 35–61; defined, 10n1, 29; importance for bioethics, 7, 17–18, 154, 181, 205–6, 211–14; in debate about Kant and organ sales, 78–80; *See also* Kant's political philosophy; and political philosophy *under* principlism; theory
political power, 5–6, 30n2, 45, 88–89, 94–95, 98–101, 101–2n1, 102n2, 122, 130, 143–44
politicization, 209–11
possession, 131–36, 155n9; *See also* property
postulate of practical reason with regard to rights, 133, 155n10
principles: in bioethics theory, 37–52; mid-level, 8, 20, 37–38, 40, 209; *See also* four principles of *under* principlism; principles of, *under* Belmont Report
principlism, 23, 39–47, 214; and balancing, 40; as competitor to other moral theories, 42–43, 57–58n22; four principles of, 8, 38, 39, 209; and political philosophy, 44–46, 58n30; and pluralism, 38; 57–58n22, 210–11; and specification, 40, 57–58n22; *See also* beneficence, principle of; common morality; non–maleficence, principle of; principle of *under* justice; principle of respect for *under* autonomy
private right, 5, 130–38, 165–66
promise, 170–72, 175, 180, 187; *See also* contract(s); delivery
prostitution, 165, 176, 177
property, 73–75, 83n36, 158n46, 158n47; original common ownership of, 155n12; rights, 78, 82n19, 131–36, 164–65, 183n40, 195; *See also* possession, postulate of practical reason with regard to rights; property in *under* body (bodies)
public right, 5, 138–43, 165–66
public health, 55
punishment, 103n24, 153–54, 179

questions, ethical: distinction between first order and second order, 16–17, 41; group context of, 37; raised by medical advancements and technologies, 18, 36

rational nature. *See* humanity
reason, 64, 91–92
relationships, 107
right(s), 105–11; altering, 162–63, 194; to be informed, 196–98, 202, 203–5; conclusive, 137–38, 157n42; general and basic, 6, 186–93; Hohfeldian, 111, 126n18; of humanity in our own person, 173, 176; 183n30, 183n38; to a person akin to a right to a thing, 155n6; provisional, 136–37, 196–97; to refuse treatment, 14; senses of, 125n4; impacted by technological advances, 141; Ulpian's division of, 183nn27–28; welfare, 108, 125n6, 166–68, 182n15; *See also* acquired right; innate right; private right; public right; right to establish *under* civil condition; rights *under* theory; Universal Principle of Right

Schloendorff v. Society of New York Hospital, 30n3
security, unequal: problem of, 134–37; solved by the civil condition, 137–38, 139–40
self-ownership. *See* property in *under* body (bodies)
self-preservation exception, 75–76
slavery, 126n18, 178, 183n39
standards for informed consent, legal, 6, 25, 195, 197–98; professional practice, 185, 201–2, 203–4, 208n31; reasonable person, 185, 199–200, 201, 203–5; subjective, 185, 200–2
state, the: basis in united will of all, 138–39; defined, 33n46, 140; institutions and processes of, 139–41, 144; *See also* authority of the state; government; legitimacy, political
state of nature, 154, 156n20; rights in, 130–33, 136, 158n47, 162, 194–95; problems in, 134–37, 195–97; *See also* civil condition; indeterminacy, problem of; security, unequal; obligation, unilateral imposition of
stealing. *See* theft
suicide, 66, 75, 84n45, 174, 178; *See also* physician assisted suicide

taxation, 165–66
trespass, 113–14, 121, 150–52, 158n47
theft, 146–48
theory (theories): casuistry, 7, 48; classical moral, 41; consequentialist, 37–38, 214; deontological, 37–38, 214; deontological liberalism, 50–52; feminist, 49–50; ideal and non–ideal, 57n19; Kantian, 8–10, 37, 40, 41–42, 71–73, 90, 188, 207n12, 211–14; Mill's liberalism, 42, 188, 207n12, 211; methods of moral theory, 106; libertarian, 52; normative ethics, 37; political, 211–14; Rawlsian, 42, 52, 57n19, 60n59, 142–43, 156–57n32, 211; rights, 110–11, 126n20; utilitarian, 37, 40, 41–42, 192–93; *See also* theories of *under* bioethics
transcendental argument, 106

understanding of risks and benefits, 185, 187
Uniform Anatomical Gift Act, 15
Uniform Determination of Death Act, 15, 21
united choice, 162–63, 161, 170–72, 182n4, 194, 195

united will of all, 138–44, 153, 157n42, 158n47, 177, 183n40, 195, 198, 200; heuristic role of, 138, 156n22; *See also* civil condition; consent
Universal Principle of Right, 112, 123, 130, 151, 154, 155n2, 162–63, 172

volenti rule, 178–80

withdrawing treatment, 14, 46–7, 30n5, 59n35

About the Author

D. Robert MacDougall is associate professor of philosophy at New York City College of Technology (CUNY). His research focuses on methods in applied ethics, political philosophy, and on laws and policies governing health and health care. He is the organizer for the New York City Ethics Workshop, a group for ethicists in the greater New York City area.

www.ingramcontent.com/pod-product-compliance
Lightning Source LLC
Chambersburg PA
CBHW020116010526
44115CB00008B/852